HOW TO EAT AWAY ARTHRITIS AND GOUT

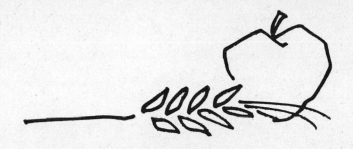

HOW TO EAT AWAY
ARTHRITIS AND GOUT

Norman D. Ford

Parker Publishing Company, Inc. West Nyack, N.Y.

Library of Congress Cataloging in Publication Data

Ford, Norman D.
   How to eat away arthritis and gout.

   Includes index.
   1. Arthritis—Diet therapy. 2. Gout—
Diet therapy. I. Title.
RC933.F646   616.7′220645   81-22468
ISBN 0-13-405647-7   AACR2

A WORD FROM
THE AUTHOR

Through using the simple dietary procedures described in this book, you can reverse almost all cases of osteo- or rheumatoid-arthritis or gout by treating yourself at home without cost or equipment.

Through the simple nutritional program described in this book you can become your own nutritional therapist. And you, yourself, can use the amazingly successful Holistic approach to healing—the New Age "medicine of tomorrow"—which treats the Whole Person instead of the just the part that hurts.

The basic law of Holistic healing is that when the cause of disease is removed, the body will heal itself. If, despite medical treatment, you still have arthritis pain, stiffness or inflammation, it is because your doctor is not removing the cause of arthritis. Instead of recovering, most people who are treated for arthritis by orthodox medicine progressively lose function and mobility in their afflicted joints.

The purpose of this book is to show you a new therapy for arthritis that really works. Anyone willing to faithfully follow the simple dietary program explained in these pages can expect to show significant signs of improvement in just a few weeks or even sooner.

Throughout the book you will find numerous case histories of people who had been crippled with arthritis pain for years and who, just a few weeks later, were entirely free of pain and able to function normally again.

For example, one 41-year-old woman's knees were so badly swollen that she had to take to a wheelchair. But after only five days, with one of the procedures in this book, this woman found her pains had vanished completely. Exactly six weeks after starting the therapy, she got out of her wheelchair and walked.

Another woman woman (62-years-old) who had suffered rheumatoid-arthritis for ten years found herself completely free of pain after only six days. After eight more days, full use of her crippled hands returned.

A 35-year-old man with rheumatoid-arthritis in his shoulders and spine was told by his doctor that the disease was progressively degenerating and within a few years he would be totally incapacitated. Yet exactly three weeks after beginning one of the nutritional procedures explained in this book, the man's back pains had disappeared. Three months later, he was back at work.

Through eliminating health-destroying foods from the diet and replacing them with health-building foods, tens of thousands of men and women all over America who were previously crippled with arthritis are now playing tennis, swimming long distances, bicycling and jogging. Provided there are no nutritional lapses, these men and women remain permanently and completely free of all arthritis pain and symptoms.

Essentially, what each of these former arthritis victims did was to give the body a chance to heal itself. By eliminating health-wrecking foods from their diet, they removed the cause of arthritic disease. And by changing to a diet of health-building foods, they supplied the body with all the essential nutrients it needed to reverse arthritis and to restore robust, glowing health.

Chapter by chapter, this book presents a detailed, easy-to-follow program for the home treatment of arthritis.

It doesn't matter how old you are or what sex you are or for how long you have suffered from arthritis.

Provided no irreversible damage has been done, such as through long exposure to steroid drugs, to gold therapy or to other "heroic" treatment, chances are good that you can overcome arthritis and remain permanently and completely free of pain or symptoms for the rest of your life.

Norman D. Ford

CONTENTS

8   Contents

HOW TO EAT AWAY ARTHRITIS AND GOUT

CHAPTER 1

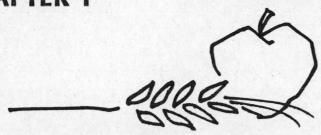

HOW RESTORATIVE FOODS REVERSE ARTHRITIS THE HOLISTIC WAY

You *can* eat away gout and arthritis.

This is the message of a new and rapidly growing system of healing called the Holistic approach to health.

Until quite recently, a book suggesting that you could eat away arthritic disease would have been considered scientifically unsound.

For years, the Arthritis Foundation has been warning Americans that arthritis and gout are incurable diseases. The symptoms can be suppressed by drugs. But the disease is always there, ready to flare up again at any time.

According to the Foundation's rheumatologists—medical doctors specializing in arthritis—the cause of arthritic disease remains unknown. Arthritic disease is a collective name for the hundred or so different varieties of arthritis, one of which is gout. According to the Foundation, no drug can permanently cure any one of these diseases.

The Arthritis Foundation repeatedly denies any link between nutrition and arthritis. It has flatly stated that with the possible exception of gout, no diet or food has any beneficial effect on arthritic disease.

But beginning in the late 1970s, a veritable explosion of new scientific information began to emerge from research institutions, medical centers and universities that caused us to re-evaluate everything we previously knew and believed about arthritic disease.

A Modern Nutritional Miracle

From such widely varied branches of medicine as endo-crinology, immunology, biochemistry and nutrition, a mass of clinical evidence became available about previously unexplored areas of human nutrition. Although the answers are not all in yet, we already have at our disposal convincing proof that certain common foods are the primary cause of arthritic disease.

Typical of the significant advances linking arthritis with a nutritional cause was the double-blind study conducted in 1979 by Dr. Anthony Conte, a Pittsburgh nutritionist, and his associate Dr. Marshall Mandell, a nationally-known allergist. According to reports, their study provided irrefutable evidence that arthritis is an allergy-related disease that, in many cases, can be treated by simply avoiding certain common foods.

The study was conducted under rigorous scientific method using test subjects suffering from both rheumatoid and osteoarthritis—the two major types of arthritic disease. Of these, 87 per cent were found to have allergies that cause such typical arthritis symptoms as swelling and pain. The study results were presented to the American College of Allergists and published in the January 1980 issue of *Annals of Allergy.*

In the following weeks and months, identical reports that arthritis is a nutrition-caused disease began to filter in from physicians and scientists who were conducting similar but separate studies of their own.

For example, Dr. Robert Stroud, a prominent rheumatologist at the University of Alabama School of Medicine, is reportedly one of many scientists to have done pioneering work to show that patients with arthritic disease respond very favorably when certain foods are eliminated from their diet.

Nutritional Science Has Already Unlocked the Secrets of Arthritic Disease

As we stand on the threshold of this exciting new knowledge, it is becoming increasingly clear that arthritis and gout are not the incurable diseases we once believed.

What these doctors and scientists are saying is that most forms of arthritis are caused by foods to which our white blood cells have developed an allergy. When we stop eating these destructive foods, the pain, stiffness and inflammation of arthritis soon disappear.

For further confirmation that arthritis is a food-caused disease, we have only to consider the results of other new studies which show that arthritis can be produced at will in both lab animals and humans by feeding them foods to which they are allergic.

Thus medical science has at last confirmed that certain health-destroying foods are the primary cause of gout and arthritis. By replacing them with certain health-restoring foods, we definitely can cause a remission of these diseases together with elimination of stiffness, pain and inflammation.

Nutritional Therapy Has Outdated Medical Treatment

These important new advances have outdated orthodox medicine's capability to treat gout and arthritis. We now have available a mass of new data linking arthritic disease with nutrition that simply did not exist when most present doctors were attending medical school.

But instead of welcoming these discoveries, as you might expect, traditional medical practitioners have almost totally ignored them. For most doctors and rheumatologists are too busy, overworked and locked-in by their own medical school training to keep abreast of new discoveries.

Arthur H. Discovers That Drugs Are Not the Only Way to Get Well

Take the case of Arthur H. whose doctor had been treating him for rheumatoid arthritis for 7 years. Arthur finally became so frustrated with his doctor's lack of success that he consulted an allergist. Sensitivity tests revealed that Arthur had developed allergic responses to milk, wheat and potatoes. When Arthur eliminated these foods from his diet, the arthritis disappeared within two weeks.

Arthur returned to his original doctor to tell about his

success, but the doctor was unimpressed. He made no attempt
to seek information about nutritional therapy from the allergist.
Nor did he refer any of his arthritic patients there. Instead he
simply went on prescribing drugs just as he had been taught in
medical school.

Medical Science Faces Backwards

Past experience has shown that the lag time between the
discovery of an important therapy and the time that doctors
actually accept and use it is often as much as 20 or 30 years. For
example, it took almost 30 years from the time that diet and
exercise therapy were demonstrated to be able to reverse heart
disease until cardiac rehabilitation centers began to appear.

So don't expect your doctor to begin using nutritional
therapy to treat gout and arthritis any time soon. You are likely
to go on being told that arthritis is medically incurable. Most
doctors will continue to say that you must learn to live with your
arthritis. And they will continue to prescribe noxious drugs as
the only answer to inflammation and pain.

Revolution in Nutrition Reveals
Cause of Arthritis

How can this plethora of new scientific findings help you
reverse arthritis or gout?

For at least 150 years, we've known that arthritic disease
could be benefitted and often permanently reversed by changing to a diet of fresh, natural, health-restoring foods. The disease
usually disappeared for as long as the person stayed on the diet.

But not everyone was able to recover fully by changing their
diet. Recent scientific discoveries have now revealed why.

Arthritis is not, as was previously thought, caused simply
by eating devitalized, health-robbing foods. Nutritional research has now discovered that food causes arthritic disease in
two distinct stages. In the first stage, the nutritional deficiency
caused by eating depleted, processed foods paves the way for a
second stage consisting of one or more food allergies. It is these
allergic reactions that trigger our white blood cells to attack the
tissue in our joints.

This explains why, in past times, some people who made a

complete changeover from health-destroying foods to health-restoring foods never completely got rid of arthritis. They still had allergies to one or more of the natural foods.

We now have so much important new knowledge concerning arthritis and gout that we are witnessing a whole series of modern nutritional miracles.

Be Your Own Nutritional Therapist

Among them is the discovery that you yourself can easily test and identify the exact culprit foods that are creating the allergy that may be causing your arthritis. You can use the identical tests that a professional allergist would make and you can do it all easily and simply in the privacy of your own home without experience, equipment or expense.

Other important discoveries show that the way you eat also affects the way you feel. Having a strongly positive attitude can halve the time it takes to recover from arthritis. Eat right and you'll feel right.

But what really swings the odds in your favor is the discovery that the more you know about arthritis the more power it gives you over the disease.

The purpose of this book is to show how you can use this totally Holistic nutritional approach to relieve the pain and inflammation of arthritis and to restore yourself to perfect health.

Restorative Foods—The Holistic Approach to Healing Gout or Arthritis

New knowledge has come from the research frontiers of psychology and behavioral motivation to show that when you change your diet, you simultaneously benefit your Whole Person on the physical, mental and emotional levels.

The still emerging rationale which is able to reverse arthritis and gout is known as the Holistic approach to health because we now know that total health is possible only when the Whole Person is functioning smoothly. The Holistic approach is not merely to ease pain and swelling but to end arthritic disease altogether by *removing the cause.*

The Holistic approach to arthritis and gout is that drugs are not the only option. Nutrition is one of several gentle, alternative therapies that have proven as equally effective as medical care.

As a result, the Holistic rationale is creating a revolution in man's approach to disease. Simply because medical treatment is the established way to treat an ailment, it is not necessarily the only way.

The reason is, of course, that both arthritis and gout are caused by our own incorrect eating habits. It has also been amply demonstrated that our health-destroying foods are also largely the cause of a whole class of degenerative diseases that includes heart disease, stroke, atherosclerosis, hypertension, adult-onset diabetes, diverticulosis and chronic headaches.

What gout and arthritis and all these diseases have in common is that they are not caused by a virus or a bacterium that could be wiped out by drugs. They are caused instead by our life-wrecking eating habits.

The underlying cause of nearly all the major diseases that are killing Americans lies in our food and how we eat it. The only way to reverse these diseases is to eliminate the cause. That is, by rehabilitating our suicidal eating habits.

Drugs cannot alter what we eat. Hence it should come as no surprise that mainstream medicine has yet to produce a single bonafide cure for any of the degenerative diseases.

All that medical science can do is to mask or suppress or cut out the symptoms of these diseases. Aspirin may temporarily alleviate the pain and swelling of rheumatoid arthritis, but neither aspirin nor any other drugs can cure arthritic disease. Yet a natural therapy like nutrition can.

A Simple Diet Change Ends Both Arthritis and Migraine for Betty M.

Ever since she was 18, Betty M. had suffered from frequent migraine headaches. At age 31, after the birth of her second child, Betty began to experience stiffness and pain in her left knee on rising. Soon the pain and swelling spread to her fingers, wrists and ankles. Based on lab tests, her doctor diagnosed rheumatoid arthritis.

Within 18 months, Betty was so wracked by agonising joint pains that she was unable to walk or do housework. Meanwhile her headaches became even more excruciating. Altogether her doctor prescribed 16 aspirin daily with Nalfon and Tolectin plus routine shots of cortisone. But nothing helped. Her doctor admitted that the drugs could only suppress symptoms. He told Betty that the cause of rheumatoid arthritis was unknown and the disease was medically incurable.

One day, Betty read about the benefits of natural foods in a health magazine. Out of sheer frustration she decided to act. She hobbled downstairs and dragged out every canned, packaged and convenience food in the house. When her husband came home, she had him replace them with natural health-restoring foods just as the magazine had recommended.

Ten days later, the pain and swelling in her joints began to subside. And simultaneously her migraine headaches began to taper off.

In six weeks time, Betty was well enough to walk and resume housework and her headaches had also disappeared. A naturopath whom she consulted explained her recovery as due to the fact that both the arthritis and migraine had been caused by the devitalized foods on which she had lived for years. When the cause—the health-destroying foods—was removed, both diseases disappeared.

We can't guarantee anything, of course. But if you already have another degenerative disease (cancer excepted) in addition to gout or arthritis, you may notice an improvement in the other disease as well as in the arthritic disease. For all degenerative diseases are caused by our same incorrect lifestyle habits. When we remove the cause by cleaning up our habits, chances are good that any of these other diseases you have may also gradually disappear.

Drugs Treat Symptoms of Arthritis, Not The Cause

As researchers and scientists assess this new information, many have already reached a rather obvious but nonetheless startling conclusion.

Arthritis and gout, along with most other degenerative diseases, *are not a medical problem*. They are simply not curable by medication. Our medical schools have not trained doctors to recognize the cause of degenerative diseases nor to treat them by therapies that actually work.

Even cutting out a diseased organ does not remove the cause. When a heart patient with cholesterol-choked coronary arteries is given new arteries in a by-pass operation, absolutely nothing is accomplished towards removing the cause of his disease.

Often, within as short a time as one year, the new arteries again become choked with cholesterol caused by the same high-fat diet which blocked the original arteries. The only "cure" for heart disease that really works is to change to a diet of health-restoring foods.

So even heart disease is not really a medical problem. As with gout and arthritis, the "cure" lies in something we can do for ourselves. That "something" is to use nutritional therapy to change our life-threatening eating habits. We can become our own nutritional therapists. Instead of cutting out organs, we can cut out the cause of arthritic disease.

Because medical science has no bonafide cure for any degenerative disease, Holistic-oriented healers prefer to avoid using the word "cure." Instead, they talk about "reversing" gout or arthritis. Unlike infectious diseases that can be cured by destroying the virus or bacterium that is responsible, a degenerative disease can be reversed and kept in a state of remission only as long as a person practices healthful living habits.

When gout sufferer John R. changed to a diet of low-fat natural foods, his gout soon disappeared. For 3 years John stayed strictly with his diet without a further trace of gout. Then he became careless and while on a cruise ate several meals of oily fish and rich meats with wine. A few days later he hobbled off the ship with both big toes swollen, hot, tender and throbbing.

Strategy for Recovery

This book is not written to challenge medical treatment. We most strongly urge and recommend anyone with any kind of chronic or persistent pain to consult a physician for a professional diagnosis.

Arthritis-like pains, such as stiffness, swelling and inflammation of one or more joints can be caused by a variety of infectious diseases. Hepatitis, strep and staph infections, TB, pneumonia, meningitis, syphilis and gonorrhea can all create symptoms similar to those of arthritis. Untreated cases of advanced gout have also caused hypertension, renal disease, diabetes and heart disease.

These diseases may be medical emergencies which, if not treated, can cause rapid and permanent destruction to joints, heart, kidneys, eyes and other vital organs. When these diseases are cured with antibiotics or other emergency treatment, the arthritic symptoms quickly disappear.

Using emergency treatment to cure infections and other diseases of rapid onset has been conventional medicine's greatest triumph. The trouble is that conventional medicine uses the same kind of emergency treatment to deal with degenerative diseases that often take years to appear.

No Cure for Arthritis in the Aspirin Bottle

Treatment for arthritis invariably begins with aspirin. As many as 16 or more aspirin per day may be prescribed to relieve pain and inflammation. The verdict of medical treatment is that you must continue to take large doses of aspirin daily for life.

Aspirin reduces pain and inflammation by blocking the healing power of prostaglandin enzymes which the body produces to help defend and heal the afflicted joint. Prostaglandins defend and heal by creating inflammation, swelling, heat, stiffness and tenderness. This is the body's own way of defending and healing itself. Thus aspirin works by preventing the body from trying to defend and heal itself.

When you take aspirin, the body never gets a chance to recover naturally. Aspirin does reduce pain and inflammation, but only at the appalling cost of destroying the body's own efforts to heal itself.

In its booklet *Arthritis The Basic Facts*, the Arthritis Foundation admits that aspirin taken in large doses can cause stomach irritation and ringing in the ears.

But according to the British medical journal *Lancet*, when cardiac patents took 3 or more aspirin a day on a long-term basis, ten-to-twenty per cent experienced dyspepsia, nausea and vomiting.

A report by Walter W. Ross in the December 1980 issue of *Reader's Digest* (page 133) states that of every 100,000 persons who seek medical attention for severe gastro-intestinal bleeding, ten-to-fifteen per cent have this condition as a result of regular aspirin use.

Everyone who takes aspirin loses approximately half a teaspoon of blood from the stomach lining with each tablet taken. Regular aspirin use can lead to asthma, skin eruptions, kidney malfunction, colon ulceration and problems in vision and taste.

The report concludes that if aspirin were to be discovered today and tested by modern standards, it would be obtainable only by prescription.

When aspirin fails to provide relief, physicians have an arsenal of other harsh drugs, many with awesome side effects. The list begins with a dozen or so NSAIDs (Non-Steroid Anti-Inflammatory Drugs) which are simply substitutes for aspirin. They are used when a patient can no longer tolerate aspirin and none of these drugs are any more effective. They simply have different side effects (in some cases more serious than aspirin) and they cost more.

The Grim Side Effects of Pain-Killing Drugs

When these fail, treatment moves on to steroids, powerful anti-inflammatory drugs but with such adverse side effects they can be used only in very low doses for very short periods. Gold salts are another drug treatment with extremely limited use because of devastating side effects.

Among other medical treatments are anti-malarial drugs which are also notorious for severe side effects. And among the more experimental drugs are cytotoxic agents, identical to those used in transplant operations to suppress the immune system. Hair loss and intestinal upsets are common among users.

To some extent, cytotoxic drugs and gold do relieve rheumatoid arthritis by inhibiting the immune system. Interestingly enough, they do so by suppressing the lymphocyte cell population, the very same white cells that have been found to multiply in response to food allergies. These surplus lymphocytes then attack joint tissue, thus causing rheumatoid and similar varieties of arthritis.

Through using cytotoxic agents on human guinea pigs, medical science has helped prove that food allergies are, indeed, the cause of rheumatoid arthritis.

Drugs—The Arthritis Remedy
That Makes You Sicker

As of this writing, we can say that not a single one of these drugs can cure arthritis or gout. A review of their various side effects includes such conditions as nausea, vomiting, headaches, impotence, hypertension, severe bone loss, confusion, drowsiness, insomnia, double vision, moon face, and deep personality changes. Many gout and arthritis drugs have already fallen into disrepute due to their excessive and intolerable side effects. To cap it all, the drugs often fail to relieve either pain or inflammation.

In reality, not a single drug in the entire pharmacopoeia is entirely free of side effects. Every single drug shows a toxic allergy response in food tolerance tests.

All of which means that drugs actually intensify and worsen the very arthritic diseases which they are supposed to relieve.

Medicine's No-Win Pessimism Can Be More
Crippling Than Arthritis Itself

If all this conflicting advice by doctors sounds confusing, it is. On one hand, we have doctors of traditional medicine telling us that arthritic disease is medically incurable and can be treated only with drugs. On the other, in total contradiction, a new breed of Holistically-oriented M.D.s and allergists is telling us that arthritis can be reversed by nutritional therapy.

These New Age physicians are also highly critical of the discouraging No-Win advice given to arthritis sufferers by the Arthritis Foundation and the medical profession. Numerous medical studies have already proved the value of the placebo effect. Because arthritis is *medically* incurable doesn't mean it cannot be reversed by the Holistic approach.

In its booklet *Arthritis The Basic Facts,* the Foundation states: ". . . the major forms of arthritis are chronic. This means the condition, once started, continues, usually for life. It means that one does not 'heal up as good as new' as after a common cold, measles or a cut in the skin. It means that whatever damage takes place may remain permanently . . . and tend to get worse unless proper precautions are taken to prevent it. It means that treatment must continue on and on."

The same booklet has these discouraging words to say about gout: "Medications to keep uric acid levels down must be continued for life. Medication controls rather than cures the disease."

Doctors in Conflict

Today, thousands of Holistically-oriented health professionals believe that this negative advice destroys all incentive to try to recover through an alternative therapy. The pessimistic prognosis given by most doctors crushes all expectations of recovery and any hope that joints will move freely once more.

Such a gloomy view closes the door to any therapy but drugs. It destroys all hope, faith and belief that health can be restored. And it effectively discourages anyone from taking an active role in his or her own recovery.

It is not our intent to raise false hopes, but part of the emerging new knowledge about arthritis concerns the tremendous power that suggestion plays in boosting recovery. Studies have shown that people with strongly positive attitudes who firmly believe they will get well can expect to recover from any disease or injury in 25–50 per cent less time than someone with a negative, passive and helpless attitude.

In contrast, the power of orthodox medicine's negative suggestions can be more crippling then the disease itself.

Health-Building Foods Work Holistically to Give Mary R. a Positive, Get-Well Attitude

The decision to change your diet is the turning point in recovery from arthritis or gout. The moment you decide to stop being a passive recipient of drugs and to strike out and act on your own, you subconsciously transform yourself from a helpless, disease-prone individual into a cheerful, positive, optimistic person in full control of your own body, mind and destiny.

At 42, Mary R. was a typical rheumatoid arthritis sufferer who had developed a deep sense of helplessness through being told by her doctor that cure was impossible and that she must learn to live with arthritis for the rest of her life. Her attitude became increasingly dependent and passive.

By the end of her second year with the disease, Mary had mentally turned her body over to her doctor. "Drug me. Cut me open. Make me well," were her thoughts each time she saw her doctor. Mary believed that her health was beyond her control and she mentally transferred all responsibility to her physician.

One day, Mary heard an evangelist on the radio who urged listeners to wake up and take charge of their lives and their health. She felt suddenly inspired. She tossed out her aspirins and abruptly dropped from taking 14 a day to taking none (a course not advised in this book).

At the same time she consulted a chiropractor who specialized in nutrition. She was advised to immediately change to a diet of fresh, natural foods and to stay strictly away from all processed, canned and convenience foods.

That night, Mary suffered the worst flare-up she had ever experienced. Without analgesics to ease the pain, the agony was torturous. But she grimly held on. By the end of the second day the continuous pain had subsided. Slowly, the heat and swelling in her joints gradually improved.

That was four years ago. Only once, immediately following a nutritional lapse, has Mary experienced a flare-up. But she returned immediately to her diet and has had no more pain. Today, she swims, hikes and practices yoga. Arthritis is just a memory.

Her chiropractor, a firm believer in the Holistic approach, told Mary that New Age medicine does not accept as final the stereotyped assumption shared by most doctors that adults are not willing to change their lifestyle habits.

As he told Mary: "The Holistic approach is that if you *sincerely* desire to be free of pain, you will take an active role in your own recovery."

Only You Can Heal Yourself

Treating arthritis yourself by nutritional therapy is not as easy as popping a pill. It demands that you become actively involved in your own recovery by making permanent changes in your eating habits.

The reason is that the body is a self-healing entity that will heal itself *when the cause of disease is removed*.

Once we remove the cause of arthritis or gout by eliminating sickness-breeding foods, the body's own recuperative powers will go to work to restore health.

The body is you. It is not something you can turn over to a doctor and expect him to make you well. Drugs cannot remove the wrong habits that are the cause of arthritis and gout. Only you can heal arthritic disease. No one else can do it for you.

Marjorie W.'s Arthritis Pains Vanish in Six Days When She Becomes Her Own Nutritional Therapist

For ten years, Marjorie W. had suffered increasing pains from rheumatoid arthritis. Life became a continual horror of drugs, pain and sleepless nights. Nothing seemed to help. Finally, Marjorie's hands became so stiff and swollen that she underwent an operation by a specialist.

For five weeks following the operation, Marjorie was unable to use her hands at all. Then her fingers became even stiffer than before.

During her ten years with arthritis, Marjorie's doctors had prescribed a total of 15 different medications ranging from aspirin to steroids and powerful narcotics. But all they produced was distressing side effects. Finally, Marjorie could no longer comb her hair. After years of suffering, she became resigned to being physically impaired for life.

Throughout her years of torment, Marjorie had always assumed that arthritis was something over which she had no control. Healing was something that could come only from a doctor's prescription.

Quite by accident, she learned about the Holistic approach to healing and about the benefits of nutritional therapy. Out of sheer desperation she decided to give it a try.

Marjorie enrolled at Villa Vegetariana, a nutritional health school in Mexico. The doctor in charge was appalled by the long list of health-wrecking foods that Marjorie ate each day. Her own doctor had never mentioned a word about diet. Marjorie was immediately placed on a natural self-purification technique designed to detoxify her whole body.

Exactly six days after she stopped eating her usual foods, Marjorie was astounded to find herself completely free of pain. At this point, she was placed on a diet of fresh fruits and vegetables. Eight days later, full use of her hands returned.

Each evening, Marjorie attended a lecture to learn how she was to eat for the rest of her life. She was advised to adopt a lifetime diet of fresh, natural, high-fiber foods.

Although she was then 62, an age at which most doctors believe our habits have become totally inflexible, Marjorie found no difficulty in adapting to her new way of eating.

For six years now she has stayed strictly with her diet of health-restoring foods. Not a single flare-up has occurred. And she has felt absolutely no urge to return to her former eating habits.

Marjorie no longer views natural foods as a hardship. She leads a completely normal, active life and she regards giving up trouble-making foods as a small price to pay for total freedom from arthritis.

Although she didn't realize it at the time, Marjorie's decision to act by changing her diet was the turning point in her recovery. Her decision to become actively involved expressed a powerful belief in her own body's ability to get well.

Are you ready to do the same?

CHAPTER 2

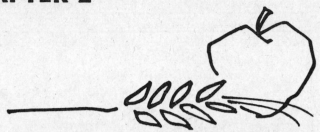

THE WONDER WORKING POWER OF RESTORATIVE FOODS

My own interest in arthritis grew out of my work as a writer on retirement. Each year for 30 years I have talked with hundreds of men and women in adult communities throughout the Sunbelt States. I soon learned that approximately one retirement-aged American in four suffers pain and discomfort from some form of arthritis or gout. Since arthritic disease is a major deterrent to enjoyment of the later years, I made a point of finding out everything I could about gout and arthritis and the chances for recovery.

Judging by the many people I met who were crippled by the agonizing pain of rheumatoid arthritis—a common form of arthritic disease—arthritis did indeed seem to be as incurable as the Arthritis Foundation claimed. As their booklet *Arthritis The Basic Facts* still states: "The cause of rheumatoid arthritis is not yet known. A cure is not yet known. . . . No drug yet developed for use in treating rheumatoid arthritis actually stops the basic disease process."

If by the Arthritis Foundation's own admission, the major forms of arthritis are incurable, and cannot be stopped by drugs, then why, I wondered, *did I keep meeting people who claimed to have experienced a complete and permanent remission from rheumatoid and other forms of arthritis?*

As part of my arthritis-inquiry program, I began making regular visits to some of the small Nature Cure resorts and natural diet arthritis clinics that dot Florida and the Southwest. And I began to attend natural food conventions. At these places, I met more men and women—people in all age brackets—who had achieved total and lasting remission from all forms of arthritis and gout. One of them was Enid C.

Enid C. Gets out of Her Wheelchair and Walks

Three years after she had been stricken with rheumatoid arthritis, 41-year old Enid C's knees were so swollen she had to give up her teaching job and take to a wheelchair. Enid's doctor tried all the usual drugs but without success. Finally, in desperation, Enid consulted a practitioner of Natural Hygiene (the Science of Natural Health).

The Hygienist instructed Enid to practice a simple self-purification technique for five days, then to eat light, nutritious meals of fresh natural foods. She was to stay on this diet permanently.

On the evening of the fifth day of the purification technique, Enid suddenly realized that her arthritis pains had vanished. Two weeks later, the swelling in her knees had almost disappeared.

Exactly six weeks after she first visited the Hygienist, Enid got out of her wheelchair and walked—entirely free of stiffness and pain. In another three months she was back teaching school.

Enid has stayed faithfully with her restorative foods and has been completely free of arthritis symptoms for over three years.

22,000 Americans Recover Annually from "Incurable" Rheumatoid Arthritis

According to the Arthritis Foundation, a remission, ". . . is the medical word used when a disease seems to go away by itself. The pain, stiffness and swelling of arthritis, even in severe cases, may subside or disappear for months or years. *In about one out of ten cases it never comes back.*"

The italics are mine. But here, based on Government surveys of tens of thousands of arthritis patients, is the official word. IN ABOUT ONE OUT OF TEN CASES RHEUMATOID ARTHRITIS SPONTANEOUSLY DISAPPEARS AND NEVER COMES BACK.

Since 6,500,000 Americans suffer from rheumatoid arthritis at any one time, this means that approximately 22,000 people achieve a permanent and complete remission from rheumatoid arthritis every year—whether or not they receive medical treatment.

Of all the people I talked with who had, or had previously suffered from, rheumatoid arthritis, approximately one in ten reported that, like Enid C., they had experienced a full and lasting remission. This seemed to agree entirely with the Foundation's own estimate that in about one out of ten cases rheumatoid arthritis never comes back.

Arthritis Recovery Secret Revealed

What was their secret? Why, I wondered, did one person out of ten with rheumatoid arthritis recover completely with or without medical care?

Starting about 15 years ago, each time I met a person who had recovered from any form of arthritic disease, I tried to find out what was different about him or her compared to others who still had the disease.

Almost every person I questioned had run the whole gamut of medical treatment, usually without any significant relief or improvement.

Yet out of their answers a common pattern gradually emerged. In virtually every case, recovery occurred when, by accident or design, each person had decided to give his body a chance to heal itself. With few exceptions, each person I questioned had made a radical improvement in living habits just prior to recovery.

Astonishing Benefits from a Change in Diet

Some had cut out smoking or alcohol. But far more reported having made a major change in their eating habits, usually by switching to a diet of fresh, natural, unprocessed foods.

Surprisingly, the majority had not done so in the belief that they could reverse their arthritis but in response to the numerous books and articles urging Americans to reduce their risk of heart disease by losing weight and eating less fat. For some 15 years we have been repeatedly told that a natural diet of high-fiber foods reduces risk of heart disease, diabetes, hypertension, diverticulosis and other degenerative diseases.

Americans were not told that it would also improve arthritis or gout. But, in practice, a surprising number of former arthritis sufferers seem to have benefitted.

In more recent years I began to meet men and women who had changed their diets by enrolling at cardiac rehabilitation centers. Actual records from Pritikin and other cardiac centers show that the same low-fat, high-fiber diet of natural foods that helps reverse heart disease may also benefit arthritis and gout.

A smaller number of people had deliberately changed their diet through reading that natural foods could benefit arthritic disease. Others had learned about nutritional therapy from friends, nutritionists and chiropractors. A few like Marjorie W., (see Chapter 1) had enrolled at one of the small natural health resorts scattered about the country where they had rehabilitated their diet under the guidance of Holistically-oriented nutritionists.

One way or another, by luck or coincidence, these people had learned about the benefits of nutritional therapy and had decided to take the initiative and give it a try.

Why There Is No Anti-Arthritis Diet for Everyone

Not all of the people who had changed their diets had successfully recovered from arthritic disease. Although all felt greatly improved, approximately four in ten had failed to recover completely.

A few years ago it was not known why this was so.

Yet today we know there is no such thing as an anti-arthritic diet that will work for everyone. The information avalanche of recent years has revealed that while some foods are so devitalized they inevitably lead everyone towards arthritic disease, each of us may also have our own individual allergies to specific arthritis-causing foods.

This is why in past times a changeover to a natural diet

benefitted most arthritis sufferers but not all. Those who were not able to reverse their arthritis entirely had allergies that extended even to some natural foods.

Due to the new work on arthritis therapy, we ourselves are now able to identify the exact foods that are causing most forms of arthritic disease.

This is not to deny the tremendous therapeutic value of natural foods in reversing both arthritic and other degenerative diseases. In heart disease, hypertension, maturity-diabetes, osteoporosis, obesity, senility, diverticulosis, hypoglycemia, colitis and similar diseases brought on by the vicissitudes of our own lifestyles, the one best therapy is a diet of natural foods.

But arthritis differs in that it is also an auto-immune disease. This means that the nutritional deficiencies caused by eating devitalized, processed foods pave the way for food allergies that trigger our white blood cells to attack the cells in our joints.

Thus a complete remission often requires the elimination of the specific foods to which our white blood cells have developed an allergy.

Recovery Program Combines Nature's Secrets with Modern Nutritional Science

When I matched my own observations with the latest discoveries of nutritional science, they fitted together like a jigsaw puzzle.

I now had the scientific information that explained why all of the scores of people I had interviewed had been able to recover from arthritis.

What I was doing, of course, was synthesizing all the scattered, pigeonholed discoveries of hundreds of people who had recovered from arthritis with the findings of scores of individual doctors and researchers and mesh it into the traditional web of nutritional therapy successfully employed for decades to reverse arthritis by "Nature Cure" and other natural foods establishments.

When I put it all together, what emerged was a simple,

workable program consisting of Five Recovery Steps that anyone could use to end arthritis for good.

I want to emphasize that the Five Recovery Steps are not "my" program. I am not a professional healer.

All I have actually done is to integrate the methods used to reverse arthritis by the hundreds of people I interviewed with the most successful natural therapies currently being used by the many small allergy and arthritis clinics and natural healing centers across the country.

So while the Five Recovery Steps program is not based entirely on recent discoveries, the methods used *have* been proven successful by the well authenticated and scientifically validated work of many university scientists and research physicians.

Chapter by chapter, the case histories I collected over the years provide living proof of the effectiveness of each of the Five Arthritis Recovery Steps.

What You Should Expect from the Five Recovery Steps

The program I describe is based on medically sound methods that are already being used with great success in a number of small allergy and arthritis clinics. Some are experimental units associated with major universities and medical research centers.

While I hesitate to say that their arthritis reversal rate is 100 per cent, it is often averaging out at better than 85 per cent. Among those patients who are genuinely cooperating and trying, the recovery rate is running 85 per cent and in some cases higher.

In cases where arthritis or gout still cannot be reversed entirely, it is usually due to complications caused by degenerative diseases other than gout or arthritis. Or, all too often, by permanent damage to the body's metabolism by long term use of such medical treatments as steroid drugs or gold injections.

However, in the great majority of cases, you can expect a virtually complete remission of arthritis or gout symptoms for as long as you continue to avoid any arthritis-causing foods and stay faithfully, instead, with a health-restoring diet.

Ralph A. Stays Gout-Free with Restorative Foods

Ten years of discussing business deals over rich lunches and dinners left 45-year old Ralph A. with sharp, stabbing gout pains in his big toes, insteps and ankles. Seldom was more than a single joint attacked at one time, and the swelling and tenderness were excruciating.

On the advice of a nutritionist, Ralph cut out all seafood, meat, refined foods, caffeine and alcohol and replaced them with health-restoring natural foods. Gradually, the hot, shiny purple flesh around his afflicted joints turned to a healthy pink and Ralph's pains disappeared.

One day, a friend persuaded Ralph to try some anchovies and sardines on toast served with wine—all notorious gout-causing foods. Ralph thought that a single dietary indiscretion would hardly make a difference.

How wrong he was! By the following evening his left big toe began to throb and Ralph was right back where he began. Since then, Ralph has stayed strictly away from all gout-promoting foods. That was four years ago, and he has been free of all flare-ups and gout symptoms since.

Restorative Foods Work for Life

Ralph's experience is vitally important. To remain free of the symptoms of gout or arthritis—as well, probably, as those of other degenerative diseases—*you absolutely must stay with restorative foods for the rest of your life.* If you stray back to your old health-destroying foods, even for a snack, you may experience a sudden flare-up. Or you may wake up next morning to find that all the old stiffness has returned to your joints.

This may not mean having to give up *all* of your favorite foods forever, of course. But it does mean you must probably add more variety to your diet. If any favorite food is identified as causing gout or arthritis, you may still be able to eat it provided you eat it less often and eat a variety of other health-restoring foods in between. Yet some foods are so harmful, they should *never* be eaten again.

As the Arthritis Foundation correctly states, arthritic disease cannot be cured. But you can keep it in complete and permanent remission for the rest of your life.

Essentially, what this book does it to reveal the secrets by which one-in-ten people experience a complete and permanent remission from rheumatoid arthritis. The same secrets promise remission from all forms of arthritic disease.

Cure or remission? What difference what we call it provided you can lead a normal, active, pain-free life without a trace of the symptoms of gout or arthritis.

Within the limitations just described, you rightfully can and *should* expect a lasting and total remission from arthritic disease.

Regeneration of Joints by Restorative Foods

As the Holistic approach to healing has demonstrated, the more powerful your faith and expectation that you will recover, the better your chance for a speedy recovery. For as Holistic rationale proves, nutrition is a critical factor in sound physical, mental and emotional health.

Provided you follow the Five Recovery Steps exactly and eliminate *all* arthritic-causing foods, you can expect the pain, swelling and inflammation of arthritis to begin to disappear. Many people have reported a complete disappearance of arthritis symptoms within a week or so. For others it may take several weeks. In other cases, relief may be more gradual.

Much depends on which type of arthritis you have. Rheumatoid and similar forms of arthritis often respond well to a change in diet, while recovery from gout may take a bit longer, and recovery from osteo-arthritis may be more gradual.

How about structurally deformed bones and joints? No nutritional therapist can promise miracles. Through nutritional therapy you can end pain and regain joint mobility. But badly deformed joints may never regenerate completely. Nonetheless, you will have put a stop to further damage.

Yet among those one-in-ten people who permanently recover from that most crippling of arthritic diseases, rheumatoid arthritis, amazing examples of regeneration have occurred.

Never forget that the body is self-healing. It wants to get well. As your nutrition improves, your circulation will improve also. The rich body-building nutrients from the restorative foods which should now comprise your entire diet are carried into the bloodstream to nourish damaged muscle, bone and tissue.

People who continue to make their health a primary concern often do experience a noticeable renewal or regeneration in arthritis-damaged joints. Gradually, as cells divide and renew themselves, structural joint damage may slowly improve.

George R. Puts His Own Body's Restorative Powers to Work

A case in point concerns a good friend of mine, George R. of Denver, Colorado. For nearly a decade, George suffered crippling rheumatoid arthritis in his ankles and toes. Eventually, his toes became so deformed that the joints spread haphazardly in all directions.

On the advice of a local masseur, George switched to a diet of fresh, natural restorative foods. Within three months, all pain and swelling had gone and George could walk almost as well as before.

But his toes continued to display bulging joints and they still spread randomly in all directions. After three years of eating nothing but health-building foods, coupled with regular daily walks and special toe and ankle activities, George's toes had noticeably improved.

Distortion and deformity still remain. But for all practical purposes, at age 52, George is fully recovered. In the more than three years during which he has stayed religiously with natural foods, he has not experienced a single flare-up.

We don't claim miracles. But if you understand the principles of the Holistic approach to healing . . . if you continue to give your body the optimal chance to heal itself . . . then some degree of renewal and regeneration of deformed joints is a distinct possibility.

The Food You Eat Controls Your Health More Than Your Doctor Can with Drugs

Depending on your doctor's knowledge and attitude, you may still be told that using diet to reverse arthritis is medically unsound.

Well, suppose the worst happens and you fail to recover. Compare that to the practices of some arthritis clinics outside the U.S. Charging huge sums of money, these clinics obtain instant "cures" by injecting massive doses of life-threatening DMSO and steroid drugs. Too, every year, thousands of arthritis patients spend hundreds of thousands of dollars for quack treatments, "cures" and devices that prove totally ineffective.

If you are among the relatively few arthritis sufferers who, for one reason or another, nutritional therapy cannot help, the worst you have done is to spend the price of this book.

In return, you will have upgraded your nutrition to where it cannot fail to improve your overall health. According to the best concensus of medical and U.S. Government opinion, you will have significantly reduced your risk of contracting heart disease, hypertension, diabetes and most of the other degenerative diseases that plague older Americans.

Of course, no one can absolutely guarantee that any particular therapy will work for everyone. Your doctor certainly gives no guarantee that his medication will ease your pain and leave no side effects. What we do say is that the therapies in this book worked well for the people in the case histories and for scores of others whose stories could not be printed due to lack of space.

Restorative Foods May Save You Money

Most of the restorative foods we recommend are not exotic or expensive but are available in the produce department of your local supermarket. Most people find these foods often cost less than the affluent high-fat foods they may be eating now.

A few restorative foods are available only in health food stores. But none cost as much as a visit to a doctor's office or the cost of filling the average prescription. Tens of thousands of people have spent their life's savings on medical treatment for arthritis and have simply become worse. Some have died.

So if all you are getting from conventional treatment is bills, disappointments and side effects, you owe it to yourself to read on and learn more about the amazing healing powers of restorative foods.

CHAPTER 3

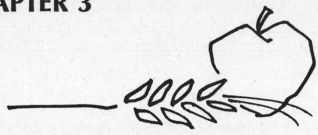

HOW TO GAIN
POWER OVER
ARTHRITIC DISEASE

Knowing all about arthritis and gout and their causes gives you a feeling of confidence and power over the disease. You realise you are no longer helpless and uninformed. Your health is in your own hands and your life is under your control.

Learning Everything About Arthritis
Helps Carl S. Make a Complete Recovery

Carl S. an insurance salesman, had suffered from severe headaches for over five years. During the summer of his thirty-fifth year, the headaches became so bad he had to spend six weeks in bed in a darkened room.

X-rays revealed the culprit as rheumatoid arthritis. Heavy calcium deposits in Carl's spine and shoulder joints were pinching a nerve and causing the headache. Carl's doctor told him the disease was progressively degenerating, and within a few years he would be totally incapacitated.

Carl's wife, a dental assistant, was familiar with medical and nutritional literature. The couple spent the entire month of August studying everything available on rheumatoid arthritis.

They soon concluded that pessimistic medical advice simply slams the door on self-help and the will to live and recover.

"As soon as I learned that arthritis was not something that attacks us from outside, I felt a tremendous feeling of power over the disease," Carl told me later. "I realized that neither drugs nor anything outside me was going to help. I could choose to recover by simply changing my diet."

On September first Carl did change his diet. Throughout their ten years of marriage, he and his wife had lived on canned and convenience foods with almost no fresh, natural produce. They replaced the cans and packages with whole, fresh natural foods.

Within three weeks, Carl's headaches and back pain had disappeared. Gradually, with much cracking, the calcium surrounding his joints broke up. Three more months went by before all the calcified joints were freed and movement restored. But by mid-November Carl was back at work. And he was soon practicing the flexibility exercises of yoga and tai chi to restore suppleness.

Still on his diet of natural foods at age 40, Carl has never felt better and he has experienced no arthritis flare-ups at all.

New Age Medicine—The Therapy of Tomorrow

Much of the new knowledge we now have about arthritic disease has stemmed from recent research into immuno-therapy in cancer. A multiplicity of studies have found that nutrition affects immunity and thereby affects the potential for developing cancer and other degenerative diseases like arthritis or gout.

Arthritis is an umbrella name for over 100 different diseases, syndromes and conditions. The majority are non-articular ailments which involve only soft tissue and not a joint. These include fibrositis, tendonitis and bursitis, all mild diseases in which medical care is seldom sought.

The really painful varieties of arthritis are classified as articular types—meaning they affect a joint. Osteo-arthritis is a "wear and tear" disease while gout is caused by excessive uric acid deposits, usually resulting from rich food and drink. If we exclude these two for a moment, all the remaining articular diseases have a striking fact in common.

Almost every branch of medical science now recognizes them to be auto-immune diseases, caused by malfunctioning of the body's own immune system.

Auto-immunity is a situation in which the white cells of our immune system turn on the body's own tissue and attack it. In the light of this important discovery, let's briefly review the most common forms of arthritis and how each is caused.

RHEUMATOID ARTHRITIS:
Currently 6,500,000 U.S. Cases

The most crippling form of arthritis, rheumatoid arthritis is most common in women aged 20–50; it also strikes older men. Target areas are the small joints of the hands and wrists and the knees; also the shoulders, ankles, elbows, neck and spine. Joints in the hands and feet may become distorted and deformed, while the knees may become swollen with fluid. Afflicted joints are swollen, hot, tender and extremely painful.

Rheumatoid arthritis is a systematic disease affecting the entire body and is often accompanied by weight loss, poor appetite, fever, fatigue and anemia. Rheumatoid nodules (lumps) may appear under the skin. Usually more than one joint is affected, and often pairs of joints become stiff and inflamed. The disease progresses in a series of flare-ups and remissions which may extend for months or even years.

In severe cases, joints may become fused and rigid. Approximately one fourth of all rheumatoid arthritis victims display "Sjögren's Syndrome" which results in difficulty in swallowing, dryness of nose, blanching of fingers, dry skin and eyes, vaginal dryness and kidney afflictions.

Approximately one person in ten with rheumatoid arthritis experiences a complete and permanent remission and the disease never returns. A juvenile form called Still's Disease afflicts children, but approximately 80 per cent of the victims recover completely.

Many scientists consider that both rheumatoid arthritis and Sjögren's Syndrome are caused by auto-immunity.

ANKYLOSING SPONDYLITIS:
Currently One Million U.S. Cases

This chronic inflammatory disease (also called Marie-Strümpell Disease) has traditionally hit men aged 20–30. But since 1970, women of the same age are becoming increasingly susceptible. It is rare after 30.

Ankylosing spondylitis characteristically begins at the sacroiliac joints and creeps slowly up the spine. Hips, neck and shoulders may become involved, and inflammation may occur in the eyes (uveitis), heart and intestines in which case medical treatment should be sought.

But, usually only the spine is involved. Typically, the spine gradually curves forward until it eventually becomes calcified and fixed in a rigid curve. Or it may become ramrod-straight. However, symptoms are often much milder. After several years, pain and inflammation gradually subside and the victim is typically left with a permanent curvature of the spine.

Ankylosing spondylitis should be medically diagnosed and any lifesaving emergency treatment carried out. Most Holistic therapists believe the disease cannot be reversed after a person has had it for five years.

Like many forms of arthritis, ankylosing spondylitis is often triggered by an injury to the target area. Indicative of the role of the immune system in causing ankylosing spondylitis is that over 90 per cent of people with the disease have the antigen HLA-B27 in their bloodstream. The B27 antigen also frequently exists in victims of other forms of arthritis, but it is found in only 5–8 per cent of the general population.

Anyone with this genetic tendency towards auto-immunity has a significantly greater risk of contracting ankylosing spondylitis.

SYSTEMIC LUPUS ERYTHEMATOSUS

SLE is a chronic inflammatory disease that strikes at connective tissues throughout the body. Victims are characteristically black women aged 20–40—the stressful childbearing years. Men are also occasional victims. Symptoms appear slowly and range from weight loss and fatigue to hair loss (it grows back later), blanching of fingers, mouth ulcers, enlarged spleen and lymph nodes, joint pain and inflammation, and kidney involvement (which can be fatal).

A milder form which involves only a red skin rash is called discoid lupus erythematosus. It often appears as a butterfly-shaped rash on the face. Full-blown SLE is a serious disease that requires medical diagnosis as well as any vitally necessary medical treatment. But as this was written, no medical cure existed.

SLE is intimately connected with the body's endocrine gland and hormone system and with the immune system. Approximately 10–12 per cent of all SLE cases are actually *pseudolupus* and are caused by drugs prescribed by doctors in treating other diseases. Pseudolupus can be produced in the lab by overloading the immune system with toxic drugs. When the drugs are withdrawn, the disease disappears. Flare-ups frequently occur when the immune system is overloaded by infections or by drugs such as The Pill.

Here is a medically proven example of arthritis symptoms that are caused by ingested toxins and arthritis that disappears as soon as the toxins are removed from the diet.

The concensus of most scientific researchers is that SLE is an auto-immune disease.

SCLERODOMA

Sclerodoma, also called Progressive Systematic Sclerosis (PSS), is a slow-moving systemic disease that strikes at connective tissue throughout the body. It appears in women two to three times as often as in men and usually begins between ages 35–55.

Symptoms begin with a dry, wax-like hardening and thickening of the skin. The skin tightens across the face and joints. PSS may spread to the blood vessels and muscles and to a variety of internal organs such as the heart, lungs, kidneys and the digestive tract. Fingers, wrists, ankles and knees may also be afflicted. The skin may become tight, swollen and dry, and swallowing may become difficult.

The first symptoms of this mystifying collagen disease is frequently Reynaud's Phenomenon in which the hands turn purple and become dotted with white spots when exposed to cold. Currently, sclerodoma is medically incurable but is fatal only if it afflicts a vital organ.

PSS is diagnosed medically by examining the blood for characteristic antibodies—*an almost certain indication that its origin lies in auto-immunity.*

OTHER DISEASES AND
DISORDERS

Other connective tissue disorders include Polyarteritis Nodosa, or inflammation of the blood vessels throughout the body; Polymyalgia Rheumatica, a recently discovered form of arthritis that causes muscle aching in the neck, shoulder and hip areas; and Dermatomyositis, a systemic disease of the skin, muscles and connective tissue which typically strikes women over 40. All are generally believed to be due to auto-immunity—a form of allergy to non-tolerated foods.

Rheumatic Fever, once a dreaded childhood disease, can now be controlled by antibiotics. It is believed triggered by an immunological reaction to strep infection—*meaning that it, too, is an auto-immune disease.*

Thus far, all these common forms of arthritis have been scientifically determined to be caused by auto-immunity, a dysfunction of our own white blood cells resulting from an allergy.

OSTEO-ARTHRITIS:
Currently Ten Million U.S. Cases

This most widespread form of arthritis usually appears after age 40–50 and afflicts two to three times as many women as men. Although your doctor will probably say that osteo-arthritis is a "wear and tear" disease, the real cause is poor nutrition. This is borne out by the fact that the typical osteo-arthritis victim is a heavy, overweight woman or a large, heavy overweight man. People become obese only after years of eating cooked, processed foods high in fat, sugar, white flour and animal protein. These same foods rob the body of such essential nutrients as Vitamins C and D and the B-complex and calcium, all of which are essential in the production of strong, healthy bone and collagen. (Collagen builds connective tissue and cartilage in joints.)

Without these and other vital nutrients, the bone, tissue and cartilage in joints become weak and easily damaged. Almost everyone with osteo-arthritis also suffers from a bone-weakening condition called osteoporosis in which the bones become thin, weak, porous and brittle due to lack of calcium.

Now when such weight-bearing joints as those in the spine, hips and knees are burdened with carrying the extra weight of an obese person, these nutritionally-weakened joints break down and we have what is commonly called osteo-arthritis. Years of inferior nutrition so depletes the bone, tissue and cartilage in weight bearing and other joints that they become easily damaged by wear and tear. And as this same inferior nutrition creates obesity in the victim, a vicious circle ensues in which increasing body weight places increasing wear and tear on nutritionally-weakened joints.

This is why the weight-bearing joints in the spine, knees and hips are most commonly afflicted. But shoulders, elbows, wrists and the ends of fingers may also be afflicted. Since osteo-arthritis is not a systemic disease, damage is usually restricted to afflicted joints. Pain is usually moderate, stiffness more common than inflammation, and the disease is seldom crippling.

But if the hips are afflicted, it *can* lead to total and permanent disability, usually remediable only by installation of an artificial hip joint. Osteo-arthritis is also called Hyperthropic or Degenerative Arthritis. A mild variety, which usually strikes women under 40, causes bony protuberances on the end joints of fingers (Heberden's nodes).

Osteo-arthritis is often triggered by a severe strain or injury or by over-use. This leads to a condition of stress in the joint cartilage—a rubbery cushion of preventative tissue—causing it to lose its elasticity. As degeneration progresses, the cartilage may wear away, baring the bone joint surfaces and leaving them exposed to grind and grate against each other.

The body attempts to heal this di-stressed area with new cartilage around the joint edges. But all too often these calcify into hard, knobby spurs that interfere with joint mobility. Small pieces of bone may break off and grind in the joints. In severe cases, the entire inner bone construction of the joint can disintegrate and become deformed and distorted. Joints often have a knobby, misshapen appearance and muscles are weak.

Osteo-arthritis is not considered to be caused by auto-immunity. Nonetheless, once the disease begins and the joint tissue becomes di-stressed, it then becomes a potential shock target for attack by any surplus white cells that may be produced by an already-existing food allergy. In this way, although osteo-arthritis does not start out as an auto-immune disease, it may become one.

Elimination of any allergenic foods should lead to early improvement. But further recovery usually requires rest combined with nutrient-rich restorative foods and a strongly positive attitude. Together, this combination will rebuild weakened bone and cartilage and gradually lead to the optimum degree of recovery and regeneration.

GOUT:
Currently One Million U.S. Cases

Gout is a metabolic (degenerative) disease caused by an elevated uric acid level in the blood. The typical victim is an overweight, sedentary male—men are twenty times as liable to develop gout as women. Although gout runs in families and may be due to a genetic tendency that leads to improper metabolism of purines in food, many nutritionists believe it is not inherited but occurs because the victim has learned to over-indulge in rich food and drink from his parents or siblings.

Each time he indulges in these life-wrecking foods, the victim's uric acid is overproduced and it precipitates on cartilage in the joints. Needle-like crystals of uric acid form and the big toe is the primary target area.

The actual process by which gout creates pain and inflammation was discovered only in 1981 as a result of a study by Dr. Gerald P. Rodnan of the University of Pittsburgh. Reportedly, Dr. Rodnan's study showed that the uric acid crystals flake off from the joints and float in the synovial fluid that lubricates the joint. They are then recognized as foreign substances by the immune system and attacked by white cells.

But the crystal's sharp points pierce and kill the large white cells called phagocytes. As phagocytes die by the thousands, they release the same super-powerful enzymes from their lyso-some sacs as in the case of rheumatoid arthritis (the process of which is described later in this chapter). From there on, the process is almost identical with that of rheumatoid arthritis.

The body produces prostaglandin enzymes to defend the joint against the flood of poisons released by the impaled phago-cytes. As the prostaglandins begin the healing process, the afflicted joint becomes hot, swollen and exquisitely tender. Gout is the most painful form of arthritis. Other joints, usually in the lower extremities, may also be affected. Meanwhile, alcohol hinders the kidneys from excreting uric acid and extremely painful kidney stones may form.

As increasing amounts of uric acid crystals are deposited

around the joints, pain becomes sharp and stabbing, while irritation, scarring and inflammation become severe.

Nature Forgives No Transgressions

If the victim continues to indulge, uric acid stones may appear in the urinary tract and eventually the kidneys can be damaged and destroyed.

The symptoms of gout are swelling, redness and tenderness in the target joint often accompanied by a low fever. Over the joint, the flesh is often hot, shiny and reddish-purple. Mild attacks may last only a few days, but more severe attacks can go on for weeks.

Today, gout can be stopped and controlled by drugs, but the drugs are toxic and often unpleasant. Steroids are often prescribed and their use may lead to impotence. Too, gout often appears as a side effect of anti-hypertensive medication. Gout is also often associated with heart disease or hypertension and can be triggered by stress.

Nonetheless, the direct primary cause of gout is a diet rich in purines which occur in such foods as alcohol, oily fish, meat extracts and organ meats.

Diagnosis of gout can be confirmed by a blood uric acid test taken by a physician. In severe cases, emergency medical treatment may be necessary to prevent renal or other life-threatening damage.

As uric acid crystals are precipitated in the synovial fluid of the target joint, they create a highly stressful condition. This stress is recognized as a shock area by any surplus lymphocytes which may have formed in response to a food allergy. In view of the health-robbing diet of most gout sufferers, food allergies are almost routine. Over-indulgence in rich, fat foods creates the obesity that leads to the body's inability to deal with prolonged exposure to uric acid. Then allergenic foods cause the auto-immune reaction that often worsens the disease and makes it unbearable.

When rheumatoid arthritis symptoms caused by auto-immune attack are superimposed on already existing gout, this advanced form of gout is often referred to as "gouty arthritis."

Sex, Age and Arthritis

What science is saying about all of these articular forms of arthritis is that, in every case, they are caused or intensified by auto-immunity. And auto-immunity, in turn, is caused by an allergy to one or more foods.

While food is the underlying cause of most types of arthritis, the disease itself is often triggered by emotional stress, a physical injury, an illness or an infection. Many researchers believe this is why certain arthritic diseases usually strike one sex more than another and are most common in certain age brackets.

Rheumatoid arthritis and Lupus, for example, tend to affect women during the high-stress childbearing years when women are more susceptible to food allergies before or after pregnancy or during certain stages of the menstrual cycle. Sclerodoma, dermatomyositis and osteo-arthritis are most frequent in women during the difficult years following menopause. Also, most women with rheumatoid arthritis experience a remission throughout pregnancy. Likewise, ankylosing spondylitis most frequently occurs in young men following an injury in sports or athletics. Too, emotional stress often sends a person heading for the refrigerator to find solace in fat or sugary foods. Studies also show that rheumatoid arthritis often appears after an infection or cold, when immune-system overload may lead to auto-immunity.

Knowledge Gives Larry A. Confidence in His Own Self-Healing Powers

Sometimes, even with the aid of modern lab tests, doctors have trouble diagnosing exactly which type of arthritis a patient may have.

Larry A's doctor could not decide whether the pains in his feet were caused by gout or arthritis. He prescribed ten aspirin a day and told Larry to come back in six months when the disease would be sufficiently advanced to respond to blood tests.

For the next six weeks, Larry suffered continual agony. Finally, a friend recommended that he see a naturopath. The naturopath explained that exact diagnosis wasn't really important since all forms of arthritis could be reversed by the same nutritional therapy. He ordered Larry to exclude all types of processed foods and to eat only whole, fresh natural foods.

The realization that someone knew enough to recommend a therapy gave Larry a tremendous feeling of confidence in his own powers of recovery. He followed the naturopath's advice to the letter. In place of his former fast food meals and sugar-filled snacks, Larry began eating delicious salads of fresh fruits and vegetables.

Four weeks later, Larry was able to walk without pain. In the four years since, Larry has never strayed from his diet which he has now come to love.

Larry never did find out whether he had gout or rheumatoid arthritis. But one thing is certain: Since he gained enough power over his disease to totally overcome it, Larry has not had a single symptom since.

See Your Doctor First

Because of possible complications caused by drugs or by other diseases, you should have a medical examination and diagnosis for any type of recurring arthritis-type symptom or pain. In cases of connective tissue disease and other less common forms of arthritis, emergency medical treatment may be required to prevent damage to eyes and other organs. The nutritional therapy described in this book is not a substitute for essential medical treatment. If you have any life-threatening form of arthritis, you should have your doctor's approval before undertaking the Self-Purification Technique, food testing or changing your diet.

The natural therapies described in this book are suggested only when all emergency medical treatment is over and the patient has been pronounced permanently out of danger.

Stressor Foods Pave the Way for Arthritic Disease

Arthritis begins with the standard Western Diet. Today, the average American derives 38 per cent of his calories from fat and 22 per cent from refined carbohydrates (white sugar, white flour, white rice).

Almost two-thirds of what most of us eat consists of just two foods—fat and refined carbohydrates. A similar flabby, health-threatening diet is eaten in other western industrial nations. So it should come as no surprise to learn that the U.S. has the world's highest rate of arthritic disease, with other western nations close behind.

By contrast, incidence of arthritis—and most other degenerative diseases—is many times lower in those third world countries where food is still produced by primitive agriculture.

Most Americans Are Overfed but Undernourished

As we continue to eat refined carbohydrates and fats along with frozen, canned, processed and overcooked foods, a condition of marginal nutrition gradually builds up. Our bodies become increasingly deficient in such essential nutrients as Vitamins A, C, D, E and the B-complex; and in such vital minerals as calcium, magnesium, manganese, potassium and zinc.

Nutrients in foods we do eat often fail to be digested and absorbed due to lack of enzymes required for digestion. Raw foods contain most of the enzymes required for digestion. But since all enzymes are destroyed by cooking, the extensive array of enzymes needed to digest cooked foods must be drawn from various organs and tissue throughout the body.

Counterfeit Foods Upset the Body's Self-Regulatory Systems

The enzyme deprivation of the typical American diet leaves every cell, tissue and organ in the body nutritionally depleted. Particularly is this true of the liver-pancreas system which stores and metabolizes carbohydrates and produces insulin. To replace the enzymes lost in cooking, the pancreas must work overtime to manufacture digestive pancreatic enzymes. The pancreas must also produce extra insulin to offset the excessive fat in the American diet. (Fat inhibits the work of insulin in helping the body's cells to take up and utilize blood sugar. As a result, fat has been implicated along with refined carbohydrates as a major cause of maturity-onset diabetes.)

When people live on a nutritionally deficient diet, high in fats and sugar and low in natural enzymes and fiber, over a period of years their liver-pancreas system becomes fatigued and di-stressed.

The extent of stress caused by living on cooked foods was demonstrated in a study by Professor Schroeder of the Mayo Foundation when he made a study of Malays and Filipinos who lived exclusively on a diet of cooked foods. Their pancreases weighed 25–50 per cent more than those of people who receive a natural supply of enzymes from vegetables salads and raw fruits.

Our liver-pancreas system is one of the body's most vital self-regulatory processes. Any imbalance in nutrition leads to stress and imbalance in each of the body's other self-regulating systems.

It can trigger a failure in carbohydrate metabolism causing diabetes. It can lead to atrophy of the thymus gland and suppression of the immune system, leaving the body defenseless against cancer and infections. And it can lead to food allergies that in turn create auto-immunity—a condition in which the immune system, which is supposed to protect us, turns around and attacks our own joints to produce arthritis.

Marginal Nutrition Leads to Joint Di-Stress

The glaring nutritional deficiencies of the typical American diet also leave the cells in our joints weak and di-stressed. Wherever further stress is placed on a joint by injury, over-use or infection, it may be singled out for destruction by our equally overstressed immune system.

Proof of the nutritional shortage in the typical American diet is the fact that almost 100 per cent of arthritis sufferers have a deficiency of Vitamins A, C, D, E and the entire B-complex. In many arthritis patients, the levels of Vitamin C and the B-complex is 50–75 per cent below normal. Again, a serious calcium deficiency is almost standard, along with shortages of magnesium, manganese, potassium and zinc. Every person with arthritis also has a deficiency of such enzymes as superoxide dismutase and also a severe imbalance in calcium-phosphorus-magnesium ratios.

A well-balanced level of each of these nutrients is necessary to supply the cells that maintain health in our joints.

Yet the foods we eat every day—the French Fries, hamburger, apple pie, ice cream and coffee—are so lacking in essential nutrients and enzymes that they create stress and imbalance in every system in the body.

That is why we call these Stressor Foods. If you listed the ten foods most dangerous to health, every one would be a Stressor Food. These health-robbing foods have also been identified as causing *all* degenerative diseases, including heart disease, hypertension, diabetes, osteoporosis and some forms of cancer.

Stressor Foods are also responsible for some of our most common food allergies.

The first step in arthritis recovery is to ruthlessly eliminate these destructive foods from your diet—for the rest of your life.

Helen W.'s Newfound Power Helps Her Conquer Arthritis

Helen W. first had rheumatoid arthritis at age 42. For the next seven years, she took large daily doses of aspirin with routine shots of cortisone. Several times a year, her knees would swell up so badly that her doctor had to drain out huge amounts of synovial fluid by needle aspiration. Helen had pain so badly all over her body that she could sleep only when tranquilized.

One day, Helen read a book by a woman who had recovered from arthritis by eating only natural foods. The book described everything that was then known about arthritis and listed foods that experience showed caused flare-ups most often in the majority of people.

Helen found that this knowledge gave her such a newfound power that she felt all psyched up and ready to act right away.

She decided that starting the next morning, she would eat only a single basic food each day such as milk, eggs, wheat, corn, sugar, beef and chocolate. According to the book, if she experienced a flare-up it would be caused by her previous day's food.

This simple technique helped Helen identify sensitivities to milk, eggs and sugar. After she had replaced these arthritis-causing foods with fresh, natural foods, her pains gradually began to disappear. The swelling in her knees slowly returned to normal and eventually she was able to walk once more.

Now, five years later, Helen leads an active, pain-free life and sleeps soundly every night without pills.

How Allergy Foods Produce Arthritis

As Stressor Foods lower the body's overall health, two things happen. First, because our joints bear more physical stress than most other body parts, one or more joints may become di-stressed. Secondly, the nutritional deficiencies of Stressor Foods upsets our food metabolism process which, in turn, unbalances our entire body chemistry. Each of the body's self-regulating systems is thrown out of balance, but none more so than the vitally important immune system.

The immune system is the body's resistance against disease. It is a network of billions of tiny roving white cells that patrol the bloodstream to seek out and destroy invading foreign cells, viruses, bacteria or particles.

The white cells can be compared to defending soldiers. White cells called lymphocytes are biologically programmed to attack and destroy not only foreign invaders but also cancer cells and any of our own body tissue that is badly run down and di-stressed. In Holistic parlance, "di-stressed" tissue is tissue weakened by stress such as physical injury, toxic poisoning or over-use.

Phagocytes are larger white cells that mop up after a lymphocyte attack. Within their cell membranes are sacs of highly-destructive enzymes called lysosomes. After a lymphocyte attack, phagocytes kill off any remaining enemy cells with their enzymes, then ingest the debris for destruction by their lysosomes. The most common dysfunction that occurs in the immune system is an abnormal reaction to certain common foods. Particles of food are rejected in exactly the same way as are a transplanted heart or kidney. Their antigens are recognized as foreign.

Non-Tolerated Food Particles
Trigger Immune Reaction

This food rejectivity response varies with each individual. An allergy to, say, milk that may trigger arthritis in one person may trigger migraine in another.

No two people have identical body chemistry. Each of us may have our own unique reaction to a certain food. Also, most people with food sensitivities are allergic to several foods, not merely one.

The medical establishment's disenchantment with nutrition as a cause of arthritis stems from efforts of medical science to isolate one or more foods which are *invariably* responsible for arthritis or gout. We now know that this is not possible. Hence the Arthritis Foundation, as well as most doctors, continue to deny any link between arthritis and diet or nutrition.

In reality, what happens is this: Every cell or virus is coated with a protein substance which carries a recognition code called an antigen. Lymphocytes patrolling the bloodstream recognize the antigen of every cell they meet as either "self" and friendly, or as "foreign" and hostile.

Immune Reaction Turns Cell Against Cell

Whenever a lymphocyte encounters a foreign invader, it immediately triggers a body-wide alarm. Killer lymphocytes migrate through the bloodstream to attack and neutralize the invader with toxic enzymes. Meanwhile, other lymphocytes manufacture antibodies, protein substances which recognize and attack the invader's antigen.

As we digest a meal, tiny particles of undigested food are absorbed through the intestinal walls into the bloodstream. When the self-regulatory function of the immune system becomes unbalanced, particles of certain foods are recognized as foreign antigens.

These are foods that the body, in its nutritionally depleted state, is no longer able to tolerate. Usually, these are the very foods we eat most of. Habitual eating of these non-tolerated foods over-stimulates the immune system, and we develop an allergic response.

The allergy that results is known as a "masked" or "hidden" allergy. Unlike other allergies such as those caused by insect stings, dust, pollen or animal danders (which produce instantly-visible rashes, hives or hayfever) immuno-allergies produce symptoms deep within the body.

Arthritis Happens When the Body Turns On Itself

The immune response to tiny particles of allergenic food in the bloodstream is to recognize it as a foreign invader. A rejection response occurs exactly as if it were an infectious virus or bacterium.

Meanwhile, the entire lymphocyte population begins to multiply in great numbers. In a very short time, the white blood cell count soars (just as during an infectious disease). Suddenly, the bloodstream is filled with armies of aggressive lymphocytes thirsting for battle.

But the only "enemy" is particles of food to which we are sensitive. With no real enemy in sight, the swarms of surplus lymphocytes zero-in on the nearest area of di-stressed tissue, invariably a joint. Through a process not completely understood, the stress in a joint somehow "alters" tissue cells so that their antigens change. Lymphocytes recognize di-stressed joint cells as foreign.

Here again, antibody-manufacturing lymphocytes produce a barrage of antibodies that will recognize the joint cells' antigen and attack it.

Both lymphocytes and antibodies then spew poisonous enzymes called "antigen-antibody complex" onto the already weakened joint cells. This toxic combination harasses the synovial membrane which secretes synovial fluid, the lubricant of body joints. It also eats away at the cartilage which cushions friction between moving bones. (In SLE and Sclerodoma, the same antigen-antibody complex is considered responsible for damage to blood vessels, kidneys and to the membranes of heart and lung.)

The Auto-Immune Reaction
Is Now at Its Height

The body responds by increasing blood flow to the afflicted joint in order to produce healing prostaglandins. In its efforts to protect and heal itself, the joint becomes hot, red, inflamed and painful. Large amounts of synovial fluids are secreted to protect the knee joints. This creates the common arthritic symptom of swelling in the knees. Swelling can become so severe that synovial fluid must be removed by needle aspiration.

As lymphocytes and antibodies conflict with antigens in the target joint, phagocytes move in to mop up. In what immunologists call a Cytotoxic Reaction, large numbers of phagocytes in the joint are poisoned by the antigen-antibody complex produced during the antigen-antibody clash.

As thousands of phagocytes continually die in the target joint, their lysosomes collapse and super-powerful enzymes escape on to the already reeling tissue cells.

The body defends itself against this auto-immune attack by creating inflammation, swelling, stiffness, tenderness, heat and pain in the afflicted joint.

This is how arthritis is born!

The Body Itself Creates Arthritis

Note carefully that the body itself creates arthritis. Arthritis symptoms were not created by auto-immune attack or by food allergies or by marginal nutrition or obesity or by anything else.

The body itself created arthritis symptoms in an attempt to defend itself from auto-immune attack and to promote healing.

Note, too, that gout symptoms are also created by the body as it attempts to defend and heal itself against the destructive enzymes released by dying phagocytes.

Holistic philosophy is that what the body can create, the body can reverse. When the cause of disease is removed, the body becomes self-healing. When we cut out the Stressor and Allergy Foods that lead to arthritis and gout and replace them with Restorative Foods that supply nutrients the body needs for self-healing . . . then the body will heal itself.

The program in this book is based on this Holistic principal.

Finding Out All About Arthritis Gives Susan L. the Power to Get Well

Shortly after her divorce at age 30, Susan L., an advertising copywriter, was struck by severe pains in her feet and knees. Her doctor diagnosed the condition as rheumatoid arthritis. His gloomy prognosis was a life of gradual deterioration on pain-killing-drugs.

Susan felt helpless and depressed. Gradually, the pain spread into her shoulders until she could no longer raise her arms. Then one day, while researching some health facts in a medical library, she noticed a report in an allergy journal linking arthritis with nutrition.

Susan decided to read everything in the library on arthritis. She quickly discovered that the newest research identified lymphocyte attack triggered by food allergies as the cause of rheumatoid arthritis.

Susan was dismayed to learn that it was her steady diet of frozen dinners, convenience foods, sugar-filled desserts and coffee that was causing her pains.

Susan learned about a study which showed that arthritis can be temporarily stopped when large numbers of lymphocytes are strained out of the blood. Another study revealed that steroid drugs reduce arthritis inflammation by suppressing lymphocyte activity and production. A third study showed that virtually all arthritic patients have a high white blood cell (lymphocyte) count.

As study after study confirmed that her disease *was* the result of a food rejectivity response, Susan realized that her life and her health were still under her control. She decided to act.

In thirty minutes she threw out all her old foods and replaced them with fresh, green natural foods.

The result was exactly as her studies predicted. It took 21 days for her pains to disappear. But she faithfully stayed with her natural foods diet. Two months later, she could move every limb freely.

In the nine months since, Susan has had only two brief flare-ups, and arthritis is no longer a part of her life.

Arthritis—The Food Allergy Disease

The arthritis-causing process just described builds on itself in a vicious, self-perpetuating action for as long as we continue to eat allergy-causing foods. Only by ceasing to eat the non-tolerated foods can we break the spiral of chronic degeneration.

Meanwhile, auto-immunity creates ever-increasing pain and dysfunction in the now arthritic joint. As the body struggles to maintain its self-healing efforts, bony spurs build up on the sides of bones and excess calcium is deposited around the target joint.

Besides causing degeneration in joints, auto-immunity affects the body in various secondary ways. In rheumatoid arthritis, it leads to fever, fatigue, weight-loss, depression, loss of appretite and di-stress of various organs. And because we frequently crave allergenic foods, we eat them in such large amounts that they may cause headaches, indigestion, diarrhea and other types of gastro-intestinal upsets.

As long as non-tolerated foods continue to be eaten, rheumatoid arthritis symptoms remain and intensify in the target joints. When a larger amount of non-tolerated foods than usual is consumed, a flare-up of the disease invariably follows.

When by accident or coincidence, one or more non-tolerated foods are eliminated, the disease dies down. It may remain in remission until the non-tolerated foods are eaten again.

If they are never eaten again, the disease is likely to remain in remission indefinitely.

The second step in arthritis recovery is to identify all Allergy Foods and to cut them completely out of the diet.

CHAPTER 4

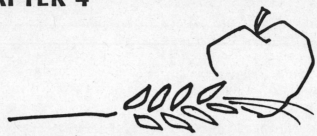

THE FIVE RECOVERY STEPS
FOR OVERCOMING ARTHRITIS

Gout, osteo-arthritis and rheumatoid arthritis are three totally different diseases. In each disease, different foods work in different ways to produce different symptoms.

Yet the basic Recovery Steps for all three diseases are quite similar.

The Five Recovery Steps

Recovery Step #1. **Cut out all Stressor Foods** (Chapters 9 and 10). Stressor Foods are those health-robbing high-fat and junk foods that create stress and imbalance in the body's self-regulatory systems. Imbalance in the immune system causes food allergies and rheumatoid arthritis. Imbalance in the liver-pancreas system causes excess weight which overburdens joints already di-stressed by marginal nutrition and leads to osteo-arthritis. Imbalance in the kidney-urinary system leads to an abnormal rise in uric acid levels, which is gout.

Recovery Step #2. **Cut out all Allergy Foods** (Chapters 5, 6, 7, and 8). Rheumatoid and similar forms of arthritis (ankylosing spondylitis, lupus, sclerodoma etc.), occur when our immune system attacks the body's own joints and tissue. The attacks are precipitated by undigested particles of Allergy Foods in the bloodstream. When we stop eating foods to which we are allergic, our immune system ceases attacking our own joint cells and tissue and the pain and swelling of arthritis gradually disappears.

Recovery Step #3. **Rebuild damaged joints and health with Restorative Foods** (Chapters 11, 12 and 13). Restorative Foods are nutrient-packed natural foods that the body needs to heal itself and restore health. When we stop eating all Stressor and Allergy Foods, we remove the cause of arthritis and gout. At this point, the body becomes self-healing. By eating only Restorative Foods, we give the body the nutrients it needs to rebuild the health of afflicted joints and tissue and to restore bowel regularity and good digestion.

Recovery Step #4. **Where overweight exists, gradually reduce it to normal** with fat-destroying Restorative Foods (Chapter 14). A return to normal weight is an essential step in complete recovery from gout or osteo-arthritis. Natural foods high in fiber and low in fat create safe, comfortable and gradual weight-loss without counting calories or feeling hungry.

Recovery Step #5. **Eliminate gastro-intestinal stress by learning to eat properly.** All forms of arthritis and gout are worsened by unwise eating practices. (We're talking about the *way* we eat, not about food.) Chapter 15 describes how to upgrade eating techniques to eliminate most gastro-intestinal complaints and the arthritic disease to which they are linked.

Maximizing Your Chances for Arthritis Recovery

When I showed an early draft of this book to an obese acquaintance who had osteo-arthritis with chronic indigestion and constipation, he returned it a week later and added proudly, "You'll be glad to know I've decided to cut out sugar and I'm adding bran to my diet."

That was all. No fat-destroying Restorative Foods. No improvements in the act of eating that could have eliminated his chronic indigestion. Nothing about cutting out fat-laden Stressor Foods.

As I finished typing this book three months later, his constipation had improved. But he was still seriously overweight and he still suffered from arthritis and chronic indigestion.

Token cooperation with just one or two Steps isn't usually enough to overcome arthritis. If you're really earnest about recovery from arthritis, you must act fully and without reservation right now and go *all the way* into *all* the Steps that affect you.

(If you're not overweight, or if your arthritis is *not* caused by food allergies, only 4 Steps need to be taken. We'll get to these exceptions later.)

But to maximize your chances of recovery from arthritis or gout as soon as possible, you should act right now on *all* the Steps that personally affect you.

How to Get Started on the Recovery Steps

The way to get started is to read through the rest of this book as soon as you can. The following chapters flow right on into how to identify your Allergy Foods (Chapters 6, 7 and 8); how to cut out Stressor Foods (Chapters 9 and 10); how to rebuild your health with Restorative Foods (Chapters 11, 12 and 13); and how to reduce weight with fat-destroying foods (Chapter 14.) You should also read Chapter 15 which describes important eating techniques that can end gastro-intestinal problems and hasten your recovery.

Skim through these chapters first to get the overall picture and to learn how the Steps provide a thoroughly Holistic approach to reversing arthritis. Then as you actually carry out each Step, you should study the relevant chapters in detail.

Which Step Should You Act on First?

Ideally, you should get at least four Steps under way as soon as possible. But as you'll probably put only one Step into effect at a time, begin with Step One. Begin by cutting out all Stressor Foods.

In Step 2, you identify your own food allergies. The recommended way is to undergo a 5-day Self-Purification Technique (Chapter 5) to prepare you for ten days of subsequent food testing (Chapters 6 and 7).

During the ten days of food testing, you eat only a single test food each day. You won't feel hungry and you can continue with your usual work. But during these ten days you should avoid any social eating where you might be pressured into contaminating the tests by taking another food or beverage.

What If You Can't Schedule All Steps Right Away?

The 5-day Self-Purification Technique usually requires your taking off at least a day or two from work. So you may want to postpone the Self-Purification Technique until a long weekend holiday or your next vacation.

Meanwhile, you can use alternative techniques for identifying food allergies described in Chapter 8. These alternative methods aren't as sensitive nor do they give as positive a response as when using the Self-Purification Technique. But you may very well be able to identify all or most foods which are causing arthritis without interrupting your busy lifestyle.

Then at the first opportunity you can still undertake the Self-Purification Technique to ferret out any remaining food allergies you may have missed.

If it isn't convenient to put all Steps into effect immediately, at least begin with Steps 1 and 3.

Astonishing Benefits from Excluding Stressor Foods

By taking Step One and cutting out all Stressor Foods, you immediately eliminate all the most harmful foods that you eat. Stressor Foods cause hardening of the arteries, constipation, gastro-intestinal problems, obesity and nutritional deprivation, and they disturb the balance of your body chemistry—all factors that lead right into arthritis.

You may also be allergic to some Stressor Foods. When you act 100 per cent on Step One, you take a huge step towards freeing yourself from arthritis or gout. Then by taking Step 3, you replace all health-destroying Stressor Foods with health-building Restorative Foods.

Step 3 actually takes you halfway into Step 4—restoring your weight to normal with fat-destroying foods. And you can easily add Step 5—upgrading your eating habits—by reading Chapter 15.

How Allergy Foods May Worsen Gout or Osteo-Arthritis

Now Steps 1, 3, 4 and 5 alone can reverse gout or osteo-arthritis provided it is uncomplicated by any rheumatoid component.

What is rheumatoid component?

Simon-pure gout and osteo-arthritis are not caused by food allergies. Gout is caused by eating foods high in purines, the basic stuff of uric acid. Osteo-arthritis is caused by the wear and tear of carrying excessive body weight.

So if you have either of these forms of arthritic disease, Step 2 isn't going to help all that much.

But . . . both gout and osteo-arthritis may weaken cells in afflicted joints to the point where, if a food allergy exists, these joints may then become targets for auto-immune attack.

Auto-immunity is triggered by food allergies, and in the run-down health condition that accompanies gout and osteo-arthritis, many people *do* develop food allergies.

When this happens you may have rheumatoid-type pain, swelling, heat and inflammation superimposed on the symptoms of osteo-arthritis or of gout.

When rheumatoid symptoms are superimposed on osteo-arthritis, you have what doctors often call "double arthritis." Both rheumatoid and osteo-arthritis exist together.

When rheumatoid symptoms are superimposed on gout, you may have what is loosely termed "gouty arthritis."

If you have already been diagnosed as having osteo-arthritis, you can easily tell if double arthritis develops because inflammation, heat and swelling will appear in one or more joints. Normally, osteo-arthritis is a fairly mild affliction which involves relatively moderate pain accompanied by stiffness rather than inflammation.

Recovery Steps for Gout

Since gout produces both excruciating pain and inflammation, the only way to tell if rheumatoid arthritis symptoms are also present is through lab tests. Rather than incur this expense, we suggest putting Steps 1, 3, 4 and 5 into effect first.

If after several weeks, no significant improvement appears, then consider taking Step 2. You should know, however, that the Self-Purification Technique will probably intensify gout symptoms rather than relieve them. This is because as the body detoxifies itself, stored-up uric acid crystals in the joints are broken down and released into the bloodstream where they immediately create gout pain and swelling.

Thus if you have gout, you or your doctor may prefer to test for food allergies by using the alternative methods in Chapter 8.

Recovery Steps if You Are Overweight

Apart from setting off a gout flare-up (which should be only temporary), the Self-Purification Technique is an excellent way to launch a weight-loss program. Restoring your weight to normal is an essential step in total recovery from gout or osteo-arthritis.

The use of fat-destroying foods to reduce weight to normal without crash dieting or counting calories is described in Chapter 14.

The Recovery Step That May
Bring Fast Pain Relief

Step 2 is often the key to recovering from rheumatoid and similar forms of arthritis brought on by food allergies. Since overweight is seldom a problem in rheumatoid arthritis, Step 4 may be unnecessary. But Steps 1 and 3 are both vital to recovery and Step 5 is almost always required.

The heart of Step 2 is the Self-Purification Technique which frequently halts immune-system attack on afflicted joints. Since auto-immune attack is the principal reason for pain and inflammation in rheumatoid and similar forms of arthritis, inflammation, swelling and heat caused by auto-immune attack often subside while pain may even end altogether.

Observations have shown that 70 per cent of arthritis pain (excluding gout) is benefitted or even ended by the 5-day Self-Purification Technique.

We should realize that it is *rheumatoid* arthritis pain and inflammation which Step 2 benefits. In people with double arthritis or with gouty arthritis, the rheumatoid pain and inflammation caused by food allergies may subside. But the underlying gout or osteo-arthritis may not benefit quite as soon.

Since in double arthritis the rheumatoid component is responsible for much of the pain, Step 2 can obviously bring important relief. But it may not end pain and stiffness due to wear and tear. The osteo-component is healed by Step 3 which is a more gradual process.

Reading for Rapid Recovery

Because Step 2 has proven to be the most direct way to benefit arthritis pain, many readers will doubtless wish to begin it as soon as possible. For this reason, it is described in Chapters 5, 6, 7 and 8 which immediately follow.

Again, since you may be allergic to some Stressor Foods, a knowledge of food allergies is a prerequisite to reading more about Step One, Stressor Foods. Hence Stressor Foods are dealt with in Chapters 9 and 10.

We explain this apparent order of reversal to avoid misunderstandings. The fact that Step One is dealt with in later chapters in no way implies that you should postpone acting on Step One.

Jenny K. Recovers From Arthritis When She Overcomes Her Own Inertia

How many arthritis sufferers will read the rest of this book then put it down and say, "I'm sure it's all very nice,"—and never do another thing about it!

If inertia and the comfort of familiar but bad eating habits is keeping you stuck in a rut, give yourself a big push and get started.

Jenny K. had had rheumatoid arthritis for 3 years when she read a book published decades ago about a lady who had reversed arthritis with natural foods. Jenny found the book enthralling. But it asked her to make radical changes in her eating habits. Although Jenny realized she was eating poorly, she felt very comfortable with her familiar foods and beverages.

"Besides it probably wouldn't work for me, anyway," she consoled herself.

Then a friend called to tell Jenny about a wonderful course she had just taken in positive thinking. The friend explained to Jenny the various reasons why most people fail to live up to their good resolutions. When Jenny discovered how easy it actually was to psyche herself up to change her diet, she decided to go ahead immediately.

"Right away, I learned I must take responsibility for my own health," she told me later. "No thing or person can turn your health around and make you well. You have to do it yourself. I learned that it's never too late to start. And no matter how often you stray from your diet, don't be put off. Get right back into it again."

Jenny's friend told her not to expect a rose garden.

"She told me to be prepared for some discomfort," Jenny said. "She also advised me to set realistic goals. So instead of changing over to a 100 per cent natural foods diet immediately, I increased the amount of natural foods in my diet by twenty per cent each week. I found I could easily live with that."

The book Jenny was following simply advised cutting out all health-wrecking foods and replacing them with fresh, natural foods. Gradually, week by week, as Jenny began to feel better, the improvement served as feedback to encourage her to continue. But despite the improvement, low residual pain and inflammation continued to linger on.

Jenny began reading more recent literature. She learned about food allergies and their link with arthritis.

"I self-tested several foods to which I suspected I was allergic," she said. "I found out I had allergies to wheat, corn and oats, all foods that the original book had said were O.K."

When Jenny removed these grains from her diet, improvement was dramatic. Within two weeks, the last of her pain and inflammation disappeared.

"That was two years ago and I haven't had a flare-up since," Jenny said. "I've stayed strictly with natural foods all the while. Once I overcame my inertia and took charge of my life, I found it was a whole lot easier and more comfortable to change my diet and feel better than to go on doing nothing and continue to suffer pain."

Recovery Steps Can Supplement Medical Care

Another factor that may influence when and how you decide to take the Steps to recovery is how well these Steps mesh with any essential medical care.

It is certainly not our intent to discourage you from taking any essential medication or undergoing any necessary medical treatment. The Holistic approach to healing does not discourage medical treatment. It simply places it in its proper perspective among all other forms of healing.

Some types of arthritis, especially those that afflict connective tissue, may endanger your eyes, heart or kidneys if not promptly treated. We certainly would not discourage anyone from taking any life-saving treatment or other essential emergency medical care.

However, when all danger is over and all emergencies are past, we suggest your seriously considering the alternative therapies described in this book. If you are still under necessary medical treatment, you should certainly consult your doctor before making any changes in diet or undergoing the Self-Purification Technique or testing foods, sunbathing, losing weight or doing anything else that might have a deleterious effect on your health.

How to Tell if Your Doctor Is Really Helping You

The problem is, however, that many doctors are so set against any alternative therapy that they will veto it automatically. If this is the case, your doctor may be doing you a real dis-service.

If you suspect your doctor is prejudiced against non-medical therapies, the solution is to change to another, more Holistically oriented physician. Choose a modern doctor who looks ahead to drugless, New Age therapies instead of one who belongs to the backward-looking cutting and drugging school.

Let your new doctor decide whether it is safe for you to practice an alternative therapy. Hopefully, your new physician will also take you off all but the most essential drugs.

Again, we urge that if you are under medical care, you consult your doctor before reducing any essential medication or making any dietary or other changes.

The solution is not to disobey your doctor. The answer is to change to a new physician who *will* cooperate by allowing you to use the therapies described in this book.

Shirley N. Triumphs over Arthritis with New Age Therapies

Shirley N. had increasing pain and stiffness in her ankles, toes, wrists and fingers. Swallowing became difficult and she suffered from almost continual gastro-intestinal upsets. After a series of lab tests, her doctor diagnosed Progressive Systematic Sclerosis.

Sclerodoma or PSS, as it's also called, is a slow but dangerous form of connective tissue disease. If not controlled, it causes progressive hardening of the skin, crippling of the fingers and increasing damage to joints and internal body organs.

Shirley responded to medication, and progress of the disease seemed halted. But the drugs produced a variety of unpleasant side effects ranging from nausea to vomiting, diarrhea and internal bleeding.

Meanwhile, Shirley had read everything available on alternative therapies for arthritic disease. She asked her doctor if she could change her diet and test herself for food allergies.

The answer was an emphatic No!

One day, Shirley noticed a sign that read, "Whole Person Health Center." Under it were the names of four M.D.s. Shirley immediately consulted one of the doctors who agreed to take her as his patient.

"Right off, the new doctor said that the drugs were only masking the symptoms of Sclerodoma," she told me. "He said the only way to reverse it was to remove the cause. He was very enthusiastic about changing to a diet of natural foods and about testing for food allergies.

"My new doctor cut my medication to the barest minimum. Then he said I should go ahead with the Self-Purification Technique for five days.

"When he checked me on the fifth day, all my intestinal pains had cleared up and the pain and stiffness in my joints already felt better.

"My doctor okayed me for ten days of food testing and he actually helped me do it. It was a new experience for him, too. Well, between us we decided I was allergic to sugar, milk, coffee, beef, pork, wheat and potatoes. He said I had no business eating most of those foods to begin with. He told me to cut out a lot of other foods high in fat and refined flour and sugar.

"So I went on eating a diet of nothing but natural foods. Pretty soon I could swallow without discomfort. The swelling and inflammation in my fingers and toes was disappearing and the stiffness was leaving my other joints. About four months after I first changed to my new doctor, he pronounced a complete remission."

Her doctor warned Shirley that the remission would last only as long as she maintained sound nutrition and good health habits. As of this writing, insufficient time has elapsed to confirm the remission as permanent. But Shirley has obviously become a completely new person with a powerful desire to overcome all obstacles and to remain in optimum health for the rest of her life.

Yet as she herself said, "If I hadn't spotted that sign on the Holistic Health Center, I'd have gone on being an invalid for life."

The Recovery Steps Are a Lifetime Program

As Shirley's doctor pointed out, she must stay with Restorative Foods for life. She must never again eat any Stressor Foods. However, in Chapter 15 you learn how you may be able to begin eating certain Allergy Foods later on by adding more variety to your diet.

Regardless of what type of arthritis you have or in what order you decide to begin the Recovery Steps, all Stressor Foods should be cut out as rapidly as possible and replaced with Restorative Foods.

For example, if you decide you must wait ten days before commencing the Self-Purification Technique and food testing, you should try to put Steps 1 and 3 into effect just as soon as possible.

If you are reading this book slowly, say at the rate of a chapter every day or two, we recommend your reading Chapters 9, 10, 11 and 12 first and acting on them to improve your diet as quickly as possible.

By doing so, you may even recover from arthritis before you finish reading this book. It *has* happened!

CHAPTER 5

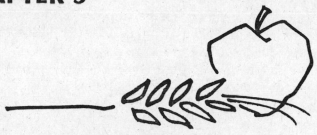

THE MIRACLE
HEALING TECHNIQUE
THAT BANISHES
MOST ARTHRITIC PAINS
WITHIN FIVE DAYS

Imagine a simple do-it-yourself technique that you can practice at home without exercise or expense that in five days would:

- End all or most of the pains of arthritis.
- Diminish heat and swelling in arthritic joints.
- Begin making stiff joints more flexible.
- Turn you into a new, positive, optimistic, clear-eyed person feeling fitter and better than you have in years.

Wouldn't you be willing to give it a try?

Well, amazingly, there is such a therapy and it involves no pills, medication or treatment of any kind.

Incredibly, all you have to do is *absolutely nothing*. The only things you need to go on doing are breathing and drinking water.

That means, of course, that you also stop eating. Well, that's the tip-off. The process is called fasting and a five-day fast is the most rapid way the the body can relieve itself of arthritis-causing foods and begin to use its energies for self-healing instead.

Although your doctor has probably never heard of fasting therapy, and if he did he wouldn't believe in it, fasting is widely used in the Holistic approach to healing.

A five day fast is also the first part of the most reliable and accurate method of diagnosing food allergies. As fasting purifies the body, it becomes many times more sensitive to any foods being tested.

Nature's Wonder Drug Ends Arthritis Pain

Fasting provides rapid relief from most arthritis pains because it abruptly cuts off the allergenic foods that are causing arthritis symptoms. But when an allergenic food is re-introduced several days later, arthritis symptoms will reappear with renewed intensity. Because of this phenomenon, we are able to identify the exact foods that cause most forms of arthritis.

For example, Dr. Theron Randolph, an eminent Chicago allergist and one of the pioneers in allergy research, has reportedly fasted over 6,000 patients. The usual fast for arthritis patients is reported to be 4–7 days. After arthritis pains cease, suspected foods are re-introduced one at a time. Any allergenic food will cause a swift flare-up of arthritis pain and symptoms.

A similar method is being used with overwhelming success at many small arthritis clinics and health resorts around the country. A consensus of their reports shows that after five days of not eating, 70 per cent of arthritis sufferers have lost all or much of the pain in their joints.

For instance, during 1980 a group of 15 patients with rheumatoid arthritis underwent a fast of 7–10 days at Linkoping Regional Hospital in Sweden. Ten others in a control group did not fast. After breaking their fasts, all 15 patients reported significant reductions in pain, swelling and stiffness of joints, while none of the control group felt any better.

Interestingly, the study was made only to test the effects of fasting. Afterwards, the 15 fasters returned to their original diet and in 2–3 weeks all their previous arthritis symptoms had returned.

Our program, of course, is to use the fast to identify the

foods that are causing arthritis and to eliminate them from the diet. So, except while testing suspected Allergy Foods immediately after the fast, you should not—provided you stay faithfully with your eating program—ever again experience rheumatoid arthritis pain or symptoms. The only exception concerns gout and osteo-arthritis where the necessity to bring your weight down to normal may prolong recovery time.

Although the Swedes used a 7–10 day fast for their study, 5 days is considered sufficient for food allergy testing.

Dennis M. Obtains Permanent Relief from Rheumatoid Arthritis in Just Five Days

Dennis M. is typical of the thousands of arthritis sufferers that fasting has helped. I'll let him tell his story in his own words.

"For years, I'd suffered harrowing pain in my hands and knees. My hands were so stiff I could barely turn a doorknob. No drug gave me any benefit. But my doctor still went on giving me routine doses of cortisone.

"Finally, the constant pain became unbearable. I was ready to try anything. So I enrolled at a small natural foods spa in New Mexico.

"The chiropractor who ran it put me on an immediate water fast. For five whole days I ate nothing at all. But on the third morning, my pains ceased.

"Now, none of my friends will believe this, but by the last day of the fast, I was entirely free of pain. For the first time in years, all my pain had gone.

"I broke the fast with a meal of four oranges. This was the start of ten days of food testing in which I tested ten different foods—one each day. Each day I ate a single basic food like eggs, wheat or chocolate. Three of the foods caused a severe flare-up. I learned that allergies to sugar, beef and wheat were causing my arthritis.

"I was advised to drop these foods along with such obviously undesirable foods as white bread, fried foods and all canned and processed items.

"Gradually, the stiffness and swelling in my joints disappeared. I stayed strictly with the diet. Within a year I was playing tennis again. And I've lived a completely normal life ever since."

Tap Your Inner Wellsprings of Good Health

But, I hear you say, I couldn't possibly go five whole days without eating. I've never missed a meal in my life.

If that's the case, it may be why you have arthritis now. Unless you're obviously thin and underweight, almost all of us Americans tend to eat at least twice as much as we actually need.

Besides, food is the cause of arthritis and gout. So what's wrong with giving your digestion a few days rest? Especially when those few days can end most arthritis pains forever.

Who Should Not Undertake the Purifying Technique

A fast will benefit just about everyone except pregnant women, nursing mothers, babies or children and anyone under essential medical care or with any of the following conditions:

Severe asthma, epilepsy, diabetes, heart disease or recent heart attack, advanced tuberculosis, cerebral disease, uncontrolled hypoglycemia, cancer, undiagnosed tumors, any blood disease, any active pulmonary disease, anemia, nephritis, peptic ulcers or any form of mental illness.

This is not to imply that fasting will not benefit these conditions. It frequently does. But complications could arise that call for professional supervision. If your doctor okays a fast with any of these ailments, fine! If not, you should fast only under the guidance of an experienced professional.

Again, if you are taking essential drugs for emergency treatment, or for maintenance purposes, you should have your doctor's permission before fasting. For drugs should not be taken during a fast.

If you are taking non-essential drugs for gout or arthritis or any other conditions and there is no risk to life in stopping them, then you can safely drop them. Check with your doctor to be sure. He will probably advise you not to fast. But the question to ask is whether there is any danger if you stop taking your medication for gout or arthritis, or for any other condition. If the medication is simply to kill pain and reduce inflammation, there is seldom any risk in stopping it for a few days.

You can safely get rid of all non-prescription drugs before commencing to fast. Tranquilizers, sleeping pills, digestive aids or laxatives—all these non-essential drugs are toxic and will interfere with fasting and food testing. Too, many people are allergic to aspirin.

Don't stop taking any drug or medication abruptly. Taper it off gradually for several days preceding the fast. This also applies to heavy coffee drinking. If cut off abruptly, coffee addiction can cause 6–8 hours of throbbing headache the day following withdrawal. You can avoid this unpleasantness by phasing out coffee gradually and replacing it with tea.

Drug use should also be stopped during the several days of food testing that follows the fast. If you cannot possibly stop all drugs, then go ahead while cutting down to the barest minimum. As you fast and pain disappears, try to reduce the dosage even more.

Finally, you should not undertake a fast if you are at all emaciated, thin or underweight.

For anyone unable to fast safely, alternatives are described in Chapter 8. They aren't quite as good for ending pain or for diagnosing allergies, but they are a satisfactory trade-off for anyone who should not fast.

Five Days May Be All You Need to End Arthritis Pain

Fasting is not starving. Fasting means that your body is feeding off its stored reserves of fat. Toxins have a proclivity for fat. As various toxins enter the body in pesticide residues, drugs, stimulants and chemical food additives, they end up in fat cells.

During a fast, fat cells are broken down to supply energy to fuel the body's basic metabolism. As they break down, fat cells release their stored-up toxins. The body then spews these toxins out through the kidneys, skin, lungs and mouth.

As a result, the tongue acquires a whitish-yellow coat, the breath and skin become odorous, the whites of the eyes may become discolored and the urine turns brown. As long as these signs remain, it indicates that the body is still breaking down fat cells and is, therefore, still fasting.

At the point where these signs disappear, fasting ends and starvation begins. When the breath and skin smell baby-fresh, the tongue is uncoated, the whites of the eyes are clear and the urine is also clear, this indicates that the fast must be broken.

Unless a person is already thin and emaciated, it is highly unlikely that the starvation point would be reached after fasting only 5 days. When you break your fast on the morning of the sixth day, you are still likely to display the coated tongue, brown urine and odorous breath and skin that indicate that detoxification is still incomplete.

Depending on the extent of surplus body weight, total detoxification for the average American may take 14–45 days or longer and require a weight-loss of 10–45 pounds or more. Extremely obese people have fasted for months and have lost up to 200 pounds.

But any fast of more than 5 days requires professional supervision. Therefore, we must strongly urge that, regardless whether or not signs of toxicity still remain, you break the fast not more than 120 hours after you begin.

An Easy Health-Renewing Method Changes René N's Body Chemistry to That of a Teenager

René N. was forty when rheumatoid arthritis first appeared in her left elbow. It soon spread to her left knee. Within months, René was unable to walk. Her doctor said there was no cure, and he prescribed 15 aspirin a day for life.

René's left knee swelled so badly that the synovial fluid had to be withdrawn by needle aspiration. Afterwards, she was placed on cortisone. But the only observable effect was a new swelling in her right knee. Both knees became so badly swollen that René spent her days in a wheelchair.

Three years after the disease first appeared, René learned about fasting therapy from a friend who had just returned from a Nature Cure resort. René decided to begin a 5-day fast right away. Although her pain was too severe to cut out aspirin altogether, she reduced her intake during each day of the fast.

When she broke the fast, she was taking only 4 aspirin per day, and at least half her pain had subsided.

René continued eating only natural foods as her friend had advised. She continued to show slow improvement. But then, René noticed that a flare-up would follow whenever she ate tomatoes, potatoes, peppers or eggplant. Although little was known of food allergies at the time, René concluded that somehow these foods—all belonging to the nightshade family—were somehow responsible for her arthritis. She eliminated them altogether.

Within 15 days of cutting out nightshade family foods, the swelling had subsided in both her knees and her elbow. Two weeks later, she got up out of her wheelchair and walked. Soon, she was climbing stairs and jumping, and she could even dance the Charleston.

In the ensuing 15 years, not a single flare-up has occurred. Today, at 60, René feels as fit and supple as she did at 18.

How the Five Day Self-Purification Technique Works

Within 24 hours of ceasing to eat, profound biochemical changes begin deep within the body. Large amounts of blood and energy are released from the task of digestion and are directed into self-healing. Every organ and system in the body is rested and rejuvenated. As the kidneys free lymph and blood of toxic excesses, every cell in the body is gradually purified. Balance is restored to body chemistry and to each of the body's self-regulatory systems.

Besides feeding on its own fat cells, the body also consumes any cells and tissue that may be diseased, weak, aging or dead. In this way, some of the di-stressed cells in arthritic joints may be replaced.

Let's not forget that all healing is self-healing. When a surgeon sets a broken bone, he does not heal the bone. Only the body's own recuperative powers can rejoin the bone. Fasting is the surest way known to remove the cause of disease and to restore total health.

While all this is going on, two events occur of paramount importance in arthritis recovery.

First, the body is relieved from the endless task of producing enzymes to digest cooked foods. Instead, the body's enzymes are freed to work on repairing damaged tissue.

Secondly, as allergenic food particles cease entering the bloodstream, they stop triggering the immune response. The huge swarms of surplus lymphocytes begin to disappear. The white blood cell count drops. And the lymphocytes cease their attack on arthritic joints.

This is exactly how a fast ends the pain and symptoms of most types of arthritis.

But unlike immuno-suppressive drugs which suppress lymphocyte activity only at the expense of lowering resistance, fasting has no adverse side effects. In fact, the immune system becomes even more aggressive in its role of protecting the body.

See and Feel Your Body's Self-Healing Powers Destroy Arthritis

Little discomfort is experienced by the release of toxins into the bloodstream. But as foods are cut off to which we are allergic—and which we therefore crave—withdrawal symptoms frequently occur.

Formerly, they were thought to be a "healing crisis." But now we know that any minor headache, dizziness, palpitation, nausea, vomiting or possible skin eruption are caused by withdrawal from food addiction.

Usually, food addiction withdrawal symptoms appear as flu-like aches and discomfort during the first 2-to-5 days. Your body will crave the foods to which it is addicted—the very same foods that produce many forms of arthritis.

So be prepared for some mild discomfort. With gout, acute flare-ups may occur as uric acid crystals are broken down and released into the bloodstream.

Try not to yield to any minor discomfort. By the end of the fourth day most food withdrawal symptoms should have ceased. From here on, your mind will become superbly clear, your nose will be free of congestion, and your senses of smell and taste will be unusually acute. Many people experience a calm euphoria free of all tension and anxiety. Depression and insomnia vanish. By the fifth day, most people feel fitter and stronger than when the fast began.

However, if any withdrawal symptom does give cause for concern, you are perfectly free to break the fast at any time. Do so by eating one or two oranges.

If vomiting or diarrhea persists, or if your pulse rate is consistently high, or if you have any prolonged weakness, headache, dizziness or intestinal spasms, don't hesitate to break the fast.

During the early stages of food withdrawal symptoms, many people do feel weak. So simply lie down and rest until you feel stronger.

Wonder Working Techniques That Overcome the Craving for Arthritis-Causing Foods

What most people believe to be hunger pangs are simply cravings for allergenic foods. You can ease these pangs by sipping a cup of hot, pure water.

Acupressure offers another way to relieve hunger pangs. Locate the large lobe at the bottom of each ear. Just above it is another lobe that covers the eardrum. Pinch this lobe firmly between finger and thumb. Do so on both ears simultaneously. Squeeze as hard as you can. Hold for twenty seconds, then release.

Now, immediately in front of this lobe (towards the eyes) locate a hollow. On each side of your head, press the hollow with the tip of your forefinger. Begin to press fairly hard. Hold the pressure to the slow count of twenty. Then release.

You can repeat the whole process two or three times if necessary. Your hunger pangs should cease for up to one hour, possibly more. You can repeat again whenever the pangs return.

Still another way to relieve the flu-like discomfort of food craving is to experience it. Psychologists have discovered that whenever you experience something, whether pain, loneliness or boredom, it disappears. So place your awareness exactly where your hunger is located. Ask yourself where it is, what color it is, what shape it is and how much water it could contain.

Keep your awareness focused exactly where your discomfort is located and keep answering the three remaining questions in rotation. In a very short time, your hunger pangs will disappear. If they return, repeat the process until the pangs disappear for good.

When to Begin

For employed people, the most convenient time to begin a fast is on Thursday morning. You can usually go through Friday without much discomfort. You can then relax at home over the weekend. By Monday, the final day, most people are over their withdrawal symptoms and feeling fine.

For your fast, choose a quiet, restful place free of disturbing noise and TV. Confine TV watching only to humorous shows and music. And don't strain your eyes with too much reading.

Avoid eating a huge meal the night before you fast. It's a good plan to cut down on meals for 2 or 3 days beforehand.

Listen to Your Body's Own Instinctual Wisdom

If you have any misgivings about fasting, try an experimental fast. Start by skipping breakfast and noting how you feel. Actually experience hunger. A short while later, skip both breakfast and lunch. Study how you feel. Then go without food for a full day. Study your body's reactions. Learn how it is to feel hungry.

Try slightly underfeeding yourself for several days. At each meal, leave the table feeling slightly hungry. Learn how you react to hunger. Then build your confidence by taking fasts of one, two and finally three days. During a 3-day fast you may find that your arthritis pains have diminished or disappeared.

Some allergists believe that a 4-day fast is sufficient for testing most foods. But the majority prefer a 5-day abstinence from food. However, if for some reason 4 days is as long as you can fast, then fast 4 days *and go for it!*

Fasting means that you take in absolutely nothing but pure water, air and sunshine. That means no drugs, alcohol, vitamin or mineral supplements, mouthwash, toothpaste, chewing gum, chewing tobacco, candy, herb tea, fruit juices, beverages or stimulants of any kind. It also means absolutely no smoking.

Barbara H. Comes Alive with Rejuvenated Health

Suppose, as in René N's case, pain is too severe for you to cut out painkilling drugs altogether. In that event, do as René did and reduce the dosage as steadily as conditions permit.

Consider the case of Barbara H., a 47-year old secretary with polymyositis. This less common type of arthritis occurs when numerous muscles as well as joints become inflamed all over the body.

At first, aspirin relieved Barbara's pain. But the agony soon returned. Rasping pain radiated down the full length of both her arms and legs. Barbara constantly felt as though she had been poisoned. Soon, she was taking 18 aspirin a day.

Two years went by with no improvement. Then a friend told her about an arthritis clinic in a rural part of the state. Although Barbara did not believe in natural healing, as a last resort she decided to enroll.

"Within an hour of arriving, I was placed on a 5-day fast," Barbara told me. "My pain was too severe to stop taking aspirin. So I continued with my regular eighteen a day."

The aspirin didn't seem to make too much difference.

"After five days, my pain had been reduced by half—the first pain reduction in two years," Barbara went on. "I was overjoyed. I cut my aspirin down to only six a day."

Barbara was placed on a diet of fresh, natural foods and told to stay with them for life.

"Three weeks later, my pains had almost gone," she said. "And I'd discontinued aspirin altogether. I was able to walk and do housework with very little pain."

Gradually, her pains disappeared entirely and mobility returned. In six months, Barbara was completely back to normal. Now, 13 years later, she feels young and active and filled with so much energy that she dances and plays tennis several times a week.

Caring for Your Body as Arthritis Fades

While fasting, the only thing you may drink is pure water, preferably distilled or else from a spring. Avoid well water or mineral water. Chlorinated or treated tap water is also undesirable. Drink whenever you feel thirsty. But it is not necessary to drink copious amounts of water.

Brush your teeth several times daily with pure water and rinse out the mouth. Each day take a short tepid bath followed by a brisk rubdown with a stiff towel.

Short sunbaths can be beneficial but be careful not to burn. During summer, a 15-minute sunbath before 10 a.m. or after 3 p.m. is ample. Keep the body, and especially the feet, warm at all times. Take a casual walk or a nap whenever you feel like it.

Keep notes on your body changes and how you feel. Any discomfort during the second, third or fourth days indicates a definite sensitivity to an allergenic food. Bowel movement will probably have ceased by the fourth day.

Break your fast on the morning of the sixth day. For example, if your last meal is dinner on Wednesday evening, you would fast all day Thursday, Friday, Saturday, Sunday and Monday. You would break the fast on Tuesday morning. It's best to break it with a test meal of citrus or some other fruit. Otherwise use melon which is seldom allergenic.

How Detoxifying the Body Helps All Forms Of Arthritis

Should you fast for a mild form of arthritis such as bursitis, tendonitis or a heel spur? Provided you can do so without inconvenience, definitely Yes. Although these non-articular forms of arthritis all begin with an injury, the injury does create di-stress. And if you already have a food allergy, it will create a constant immune response with surplus lymphocytes ready to harass the injured bursa, tendon or heel fascia.

Even if you don't have any form of arthritis at all, it's best to eliminate any food allergies you can identify. For auto-immunity can cause other illnesses besides arthritis or gout.

During a 5-day fast, you may easily lose 5–10 pounds. Much fluid is expelled and weight-loss is rapid. When you break the fast, you will replace the fluid. But the fat you lost does not have to be replaced. If you are overweight and especially if you have osteo-arthritis or gout, a five day fast is a splendid way to launch a weight-reducing program. As you progress to a diet of Restorative Foods, your weight will gradually reach its optimum level without further dieting. For more about losing weight, see Chapter 14.

It's Easy to Stop Smoking During Detoxification

You can use a fast as an easy way to stop smoking. Tobacco smoke is such a powerful allergen that it always tests out as positive for *everyone* in *every* kind of allergy test.

That is why smoking is not permitted during a fast. Even if it were, you would find smoking extremely unattractive on an empty stomach. If you did get the urge to smoke during a fast and actually lit up, the result would be highly unsatisfying. People who light up again after a five day fast report that their cigarettes taste like poison.

As a result, tobacco withdrawal symptoms simply mingle with food withdrawal symptoms during a fast.

Since it takes only 5 days for complete physical withdrawal from tobacco addiction, when you break your fast you will already have broken all physical dependence on nicotine. You will have absolutely no further physical need for cigarettes, pipes or cigars.

So during the fast, visualize yourself as starting out on an exciting new life as a non-smoker. Throw away any cigarettes, pipes or cigars, lighters, pouches or any other smoking paraphernalia.

Even when the fast ends, you must not begin to smoke again while food allergy testing is in progress. That can occupy up to ten additional days. So seize the opportunity and begin a new life free of both nicotine and arthritis. At no other point in life is it as easy to quit altogether as when you break a fast.

Becoming a non-smoker is undoubtedly the greatest single step anyone can take towards improving his or her health and adding years to his or her life. Because giving up smoking relieves the immune system of such a heavy overload of allergenic tars and nicotine, many people find that their arthritis or gout improves significantly when they become non-smokers. Sometimes arthritis disappears altogether.

Special Self-Healing Hints for
Gout and Osteo-Arthritis

What if you fast five full days and still have arthritis pains?

First, if you have gout, the pains are likely to continue or even to flare up during the fast. This is because while fasting, the body continues to break down uric acid crystals in the joints. The uric acid then enters the bloodstream causing a continuation of gout symptoms.

Eventually, if you continued to fast, all uric acid deposits would be broken down and excreted. But that might take 2–3 weeks or even longer in an obese person.

If gout persists, simply break the fast on the sixth morning and go on with your planned food allergy tests. Low level pain may continue. But any allergenic food will produce an unmistakable flare-up. Once you eliminate these Allergy Foods along with Stressor Foods that produce gout (see Chapter 10), the pain and symptoms of gout will gradually disappear.

The only other condition in which pain may continue after fasting for 5 full days is when a person has osteo-arthritis in which there is no auto-immune reaction. Excluding gout, almost all cases in which pain continues after fasting 5 full days involve osteo-arthritis caused solely by physical wear and tear. In this case, the remedy is almost always to bring weight back down to normal so that the afflicted joints are relieved of the stress of carrying the excess weight. Having come this far, though, a person with unrelieved osteo-arthritis pain may just as well continue on with the planned food allergy tests. Even if no allergy response is found, this knowledge is extremely helpful in planning for recovery.

The food allergy tests which begin immediately when you break the fast are described in Chapters 6 and 7.

CHAPTER 6

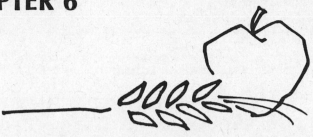

ALLERGY FOODS THAT TRIGGER ARTHRITIC DISEASE

Before fasting—as far in advance as possible—start making a list of foods that you normally eat and to which you suspect you may be allergic. (Throughout this chapter and the remainder of this book, when we mention food it also implies beverages or drinks of all kinds.)

You May Be Addicted to an Arthritis-Causing Food

Any food to which you are addicted is probably allergenic. Many people are addicted to such foods as wheat, bread, sugar, soft drinks, milk, chocolate and coffee. If they do not get these foods regularly, they experience such withdrawal symptoms as feeling weak and tired.

As soon as they eat the addictive food once more, they feel good again. So be extremely suspicious of any food that gives you a lift. Most of us don't realize we are addicted to such foods because we always give ourselves a fix—meaning we eat more of the food—as soon as we feel the need. So we continue to eat large quantities of a relatively few foods to which we are addicted. We often eat these same foods several times each day.

Be suspicious of any food that you eat frequently in large

amounts. This caution may even apply to whole, natural health-building foods.

While many food allergens are found among health-destroying Stressor Foods which are bad for everybody, we may also develop an allergy to a food such as citrus or lettuce that for most people is considered a desirable, health-restoring food.

Whenever, through poor nutrition, our body becomes run down, it can develop an intolerance for any food which we eat a lot of. That same food can then trigger the auto-immune reaction that causes rheumatoid arthritis.

How to Identify a Food Addiction

Whenever a food to which we are addicted is omitted from a meal, we begin to experience vague discomfort. The meal seems incomplete. Actually, we are experiencing withdrawal symptoms that can turn into headaches, abdominal cramps, emotional stress, muscle ache, fatigue, or lack of energy and similar flu-like discomforts.

Answering the following questions can help uncover hidden food allergies. Answer each question by naming the foods concerned and remember that food includes beverages.

1. What food would you miss most if it were no longer available?

2. Must you eat any particular food the last thing at night in order to sleep?

3. Must you eat any specific food before you are able to face the day?

4. Must you eat any specific foods at lunch or during snack time?

5. Must you eat any specific food such as bread, potatoes, milk, eggs or corn in some form at every meal?

6. Do you always stock up on certain specific foods because of a compulsive fear of running out?

7. Is any meal incomplete without a specific food?

8. Are you uncomfortable if you miss a meal, or are late for a meal, containing certain foods?

9. Would the discomfort be relieved if you ate the food?

10. Does eating a certain food always seem to be followed by a flare-up of gout or arthritis?

11. Does eating a large quantity of any food always seem to be followed by a flare-up of arthritis symptoms?

12. Does eating any food invariably cause indigestion, heartburn, gas or gastro-intestinal trouble of any sort?

Joan B's Arthritis Disappears When She Unmasks Her Hidden Food Addictions

How well can the preceding questions help you identify arthritis-causing foods?

Similar self-inquiry certainly helped Joan B. who, for 4 years, had suffered agonizing pains for rheumatoid arthritis in her hands and left knee. Her doctor had tried a whole arsenal of drugs on her without success. But let Joan tell her own story.

"All the drugs did was to worsen the abdominal cramps and diarrhea I'd been suffering from for years. Together with the arthritis, it was all so bad I had to give up my typing job to stay home and rest.

"Then in 1978 I read in a medical journal that addiction to common foods was suspected as the cause of rheumatoid arthritis. I knew nothing of fasting or food testing at the time. But I decided to phase out my drugs and to go ahead and do something about my arthritis on my own.

"So I analyzed my eating habits. I strongly suspected I was addicted to bread, sugar, tomatoes, hamburger and coffee. I went right ahead and just cut out those foods completely.

"I did feel slightly uncomfortable for a few days without my favorite foods. But after a week, the arthritis began to improve, quite noticeably. And for the first time in years, my digestive pains cleared up completely.

"I still had low level arthritis pain and stiffness. But I was really elated with my success. So I consulted an M.D., who specialized in allergies. He congratulated me and said I had probably uncovered a masked addiction to all of the foods I suspected.

"Just to be sure, though, he put me on a purifying fast, then had me eat test meals of wheat, rye, yeast, sugar, tomatoes, hamburger and coffee.

"I tested allergy-positive to wheat, sugar, hamburger and coffee. But I'm still able to eat rye, yeast and tomatoes. I'd never have known this without fasting and food testing. I'd have gone on avoiding rye, yeast and tomatoes unnecessarily."

Although some deformity remains, Joan has recovered much of the mobility in her hands and knee. She can still not type, but loves her new job as a receptionist. Today she leads an active and completely normal life.

Why We Don't Need to Test Stressor Foods

As you read in Chapter 3, the body develops food allergies as a result of marginal nutrition. People who enjoy optimum nutrition do not develop food sensitivities nor do they suffer from arthritis or gout. By contrast, virtually everyone with arthritis or gout suffers from a serious nutritional deficiency.

To recover from gout or arthritis, we must cut out all Stressor Foods—those health-destroying foods that nutritionally deplete the body and create physical stress—and replace these bad foods with health-building Restorative Foods.

But it takes time to rebuild a run-down body and to restore the damage done by years of wrong eating. Which is why our *immediate* goal is to identify and phase out those allergenic foods that actually trigger rheumatoid arthritis.

Nonetheless, if you hope to become permanently free of arthritis or gout, you should put Recovery Steps 1 and 3 into effect immediately. That is, you should cut out all Stressor Foods and replace them with Restorative Foods.

You'll find a complete list of all Stressor Foods in Chapter 10. But here is a brief list:

FAT: hydrogenated vegetable oils; saturated fats—butter, lard, all fatty meats; seafood and shellfish; eggs.

COW'S MILK AND MILK PRODUCTS: homogenized and pasteurized whole milk, cream, sour cream, cream cheese, hard cheese.

ORGAN MEATS: sweetbreads, brains, kidneys, hearts, liver, tongue; includes fish roe

ALCOHOL: all liquor, beer and wine.

CAFFEINE: coffee, tea, chocolate, cocoa, cola drinks.

REFINED CARBOHYDRATES: sugar, white flour, hulled rice and all refined flours and cereals. Soft drinks; all breads unless made completely with 100 per cent whole grain flour and containing no sugar, fat or additives.

SWEETENERS: saccharine, fructose or any synthetic or artificial sweetener. Any food or drink containing sugar or any sweetener listed here.

CONDIMENTS: mayonnaise, commercial sauces, MSG, hot spices, pepper, salt.

PROCESSED FOODS: any packaged, processed, convenience, canned, pre-cooked, manufactured, prepared, artificial, substitute or fast food. Includes sausages, luncheon meats and smoked meats or fish; also all baked goods.

ADDITIVES, CHEMICALS: any food containing chemicals or additives.

Any food product containing one or more Stressor Foods must be considered equally tabu. The list extends to practically every food carried on supermarket shelves.

Now since you will not be eating any of these foods ever again at any time in your life, it is superfluous to spend time testing any Stressor Food. Hence in the list of common allergenic foods that follow, all Stressor Foods are marked with an asterisk. And it is assumed that you will not want to test them because you will never be eating them again.

Only Basic Foods Should Be Tested

A basic food is something like wheat, sugar, soybeans, coffee, milk or corn which cannot be broken down into any component foods. For instance, most breads are not basic foods. They may contain wheat, rye, sugar, yeast, soy oil, shortening and other basic foods. Only unleavened bread made of flour and water and nothing else could be considered a basic food.

Thus any item such as lasagna, mayonnaise, hot cakes, fried foods, soft drinks, or ice cream that contains more than a single basic food must be tested by separately testing each ingredient. If you suspect hamburgers, for instance, your sensitivity may be to the wheat, sugar or yeast in the roll or to the meat itself. With bread, you may be sensitive only to yeast and not to any of the other ingredients. With fried foods, you may be allergic to the food itself or to the fat it is fried in.

Therefore only basic foods should be tested. And each basic food must be tested separately.

(If for some special reason you do wish to test a non-basic food such as commercial bread or a Stressor Food like canned ham, sugar or hamburger, the test procedure is the same as for basic foods. However, you will not be able to identify exactly which ingredient of bread is the real culprit. And since Stressor Foods create the condition of nutritional stress which precedes arthritic disease, you should not be eating these health-wrecking foods at all.)

Foods You Crave Often Cause Arthritis

The next step is to break down your list into basic foods. Head your list with the basic foods you crave most of, eat most often and eat the largest amounts of. Then add the remainder in decreasing order. (*These are also Stressor Foods.)

A typical list might read like this:

Wheat	*Pork and bacon
*Milk and cheese	Chicken
*Eggs	Lamb
*Sugar	Oats
*Beef	Brown rice
*Coffee	Soybeans and soy products
*Chocolate	Honey
Veal	Peanuts
*Tongue	Tomatoes
*Canned tunafish	Lettuce
Oranges	

The Foods That Cause Arthritis

To give you a better idea of foods to which you may have a hidden allergy, here are lists of the most common, fairly common, and less common foods that cause rheumatoid arthritis.

Statistically you are most likely to have an allergy to such foods as sugar, wheat, milk, beef, rye, caffeine, eggs, pork and chocolate. But every person has his own unique body chemistry. You may find you have no sensitivity at all to any of the most common allergy foods but a reaction to one or more foods in the "fairly common" or "less common" groups.

In each group, the most common arthritis-causing allergens are listed first, others in descending order. Those marked with an asterisk are also Stressor Foods.

Most Common Allergens

Drugs
Tobacco smoke
*Alcohol and wine
*Sugar and candy
Wheat (and products including bread)
*Cows' milk
*Beef
Rye
*Coffee and tea
*Eggs
*Pork
*Chocolate
Yeast (bakers and/or brewers)

Chicken
*Soft drinks
*Hot dogs
*Bacon
*Tongue
*Sausage and smoked meats
*Cheese
*Mayonnaise
*MSG
*Vinegar
*Pepper
*Hot spices
*Canned tunafish

Fairly Common Allergens

*Lamb and mutton
*Veal
Oats
Corn
Potatoes
Oranges
Carrots
Tomatoes

Apples
Lettuce
Soybeans and soy products
Peanuts
Green beans
Spinach
Cottage Cheese
Yogurt

Less Common Allergens

Apricots
Peaches
Berries
Pineapples
Cucumbers
Green peppers
Asparagus

Honey
Mushrooms
Coconut
Onion
Rice
Nuts

Usually, if you have a sensitivity to soy, wheat, rye, corn or similar foods from which other products are made, you will be sensitive to these other food products also. But with milk, this is not always true. People with a sensitivity to milk, cream and hard cheese may not be sensitive to cottage cheese or yogurt. So it may be necessary to test milk products separately.

Again, only homogenized milk is usually allergenic. Raw milk and all raw milk products are usually well tolerated. Cow's milk is the principal culprit. Goat's milk seldom produces allergies.

A Severe Case of Arthritis Ends
When Allergy Foods Are Dropped

Can less common forms of arthritis be helped by eliminating allergenic foods?

Richard A. a 28-year old accountant, was diagnosed by X-rays as having ankylosing spondylitis. Since the onset of his disease, Richard had become a great believer in natural healing and was well acquainted with fasting and nutritional therapy. Fortunately, Richard's doctor was also personally interested in allergy and nutritional therapy and he agreed to cooperate in reversing Richard's arthritis without drugs.

Because one person in four with ankylosing spondylitis is afflicted with inflammation of the eyes, Richard's doctor recommended maintaining minimum medication to prevent eye inflammation. The doctor gave Richard his blessing and took him off all aspirin and other non-essential drugs.

Richard immediately began a 5-day fast. The pain and inflammation in his lower spine and legs began to decrease. But when he broke the fast with a slice of melon, low-level back pains still smouldered on. His doctor said they were caused by the maintenance drugs. Even so, Richard felt sure he could recognize a flare-up caused by any food sensitivity.

Richard's doctor instructed him to test one new food each day. The foods, of course, were common allergens. Both sugar and wheat produced severe pain in his sacroiliac. Milk brought pain and stiffness in his lower back and legs. Beef left him feeling tired and his spine felt poker-stiff.

These foods were dropped immediately and were replaced with whole, fresh natural foods and produce. Richard's ankylosing spondylitis didn't disappear overnight. But over the next six months he gradually became so free of arthritis symptoms that his doctor took him off all medication.

It's too early to tell whether Richard's remission is permanent. But his back is neither rigid nor fused in a curve—the usual end results of ankylosing spondylitis—and he was recently still free of all arthritis symptoms.

The Foods You Test
Must Have Been Eaten Recently

When your list of suspected basic foods is complete, check to be sure that you actually eat all of these at least once or twice during the five days preceding your fast.

This is because when you stop eating a non-tolerated food, your sensitivity to it increases sharply for the next several days. If you eat an allergenic food after having abstained from it for, say, three or four days, it will produce a sharply magnified reaction.

But after a week or more has gone by without the food, the immune system often begins to lose antibodies to that specific food. So after abstaining from a food for, say, several weeks, that food may no longer test out as allergenic.

For a non-tolerated food to show an allergenic response, it should be eaten at least once or twice in the five days preceding your fast. (The same applies when using any alternative method of food testing.)

The Self-Purification Technique
Magnifies Food Sensitivity

During the first few days after breaking the fast, the foods you eat have a tremendously magnified power to cause arthritis symptoms. If they are allergenic, the first few foods you eat may produce symptoms of arthritis or other discomfort in just a few hours or possibly less. But the power of this reaction gradually diminishes. Thus we suggest testing foods for not longer than ten days following the end of your fast.

We Lose Sensitivity to Foods
When We Stop Eating Them

If you abstain from a non-tolerated food while eating normally, you would probably lose most sensitivity to that food within two weeks or so.

But the sensitivity quickly returns when you begin to eat the food regularly again. For example, if you abstained from a food for six weeks, then ate it once, you would probably experience no reaction. But that single exposure would suffice for your immune system to build fresh antibodies. If you then began eating the food every day, or every second or third day, the original sensitivity would rapidly return.

We Can Often Eat Allergy Foods Again if We Add Variety to Our Diet

Regardless how long you live, Stressor Foods should never be eaten again. But as you replace Stressor Foods with Restorative Foods, and your body begins to regain its health, you very probably can begin to eat some of your favorite Allergy Foods again.

For example, if after abstaining for six-to-eight weeks or more, you begin to eat a non-tolerated food only at well-spaced-out intervals, the original sensitivity often does not build up to its former intensity. By adding variety to your diet and spacing out the occasions on which you eat previously-allergenic foods, you may very well be able to continue to enjoy them.

Foods that you can eat again on a rotating basis after a period of abstinence are known as *cyclical* allergens.

However, some foods *always* set off a reaction. Regardless how long you abstain or how little you eat, every time you eat that food a flare-up follows. Such foods are called *fixed* reaction allergens and their antibodies seem to remain in the bloodstream indefinitely. When, after an abstinence, the food is eaten again, a flare-up of arthritis symptoms soon follows.

Leonard K's Mysterious Weekend Arthritis

Flare-ups are often set off when a person who has changed to a health-restoring diet lapses and goes on an eating binge of allergenic foods. Even though only one of the foods is a fixed reaction allergen, this is sufficient to trigger a painful flare-up of arthritis pain and swelling.

Leonard K., a stockbroker friend of mine, has a flare-up of rheumatoid arthritis regularly every Sunday and Monday. The pain and inflammation gradually die away by the following Friday.

About a year ago, Leonard had, at my suggestion, undergone a fast and food tests. He had carefully dropped all allergy-positive foods from his diet along with most Stressor Foods. Within a few weeks, the rheumatoid arthritis pain in his ankles and knees had subsided and he seemed well on the way to recovery.

Then something went wrong. Every weekend, Leonard's pain and inflammation returned. And though it gradually diminished during the week, it never had a chance to really get better. Because the following weekend, Leonard experienced still another flare-up.

"You're eating something you shouldn't," I told him.

"Absolutely not," Leonard said, "come to dinner Saturday night and see."

Leonard's statement was literally true. But in nutritional therapy, food means everything we take into our mouths including smoke, drugs and beverages.

During the evening, Leonard sipped his way through at least four generous tumblers of Bourbon on the rocks.

"There's your trouble," I said. "Alcohol is a fixed reaction allergen. Cut out the liquor and your arthritis will disappear."

"I've decided not to," Leonard said. "The comfort I get from drinking on weekend nights is greater than the discomfort of arthritis during the week."

The moral here is that learning which foods cause your arthritis does not stop the disease. To overcome arthritis you have to cut these foods and drinks out of your diet—and keep them out.

Testing One Food at a Time

Each food on your list should be tested by eating a normal-sized meal composed entirely of that food. And you should eat three meals of that food in one day.

Next day, you repeat the same thing with the next food to be tested. Since you can continue testing for ten days after breaking the fast, this allows you to test ten different foods.

Now, ten basic foods may not seem many. But, remember, you don't need to test any Stressor Foods.

Let's return for a moment to the list of typical suspect foods given earlier. Of these 21 foods, 9 carried an asterisk showing they were Stressor Foods and need not be tested. Hence only 12 foods required testing. And as lists go, this one was unusually long.

If you do have more than ten foods to test, here's how to handle it. Test the ten foods that you suspect most at the rate of one per day. Then check out the remainder with the alternative tests described in Chapter 8.

Using our same list of suspect foods, here's how your ten day test-meal schedule might look:

Monday: oranges   Saturday: lamb
Tuesday: chicken   Sunday: brown rice
Wednesday: wheat   Monday: soybeans and soy
                               products
Thursday: veal   Tuesday: tomatoes
Friday: oats   Wednesday: peanuts

For reasons discussed below, we chose to test oranges the first day. Honey and lettuce were left for testing later by an alternative method.

Which Food to Test First

We'd suggest breaking the fast with a piece of melon which is seldom allergenic. However, if you're going to test any fruit, you could break the fast with a meal of this fruit (such as oranges) and continue to test that fruit for the remainder of the first day.

Since as you break the fast your body will greatly magnify any allergy effects, avoid a large first meal. If you decide on oranges, two or three normal-sized oranges should be sufficient for the first meal.

Otherwise, break the fast with a slice or two of melon and a couple of hours later, eat your first test meal. Begin by testing the food you suspect most and work down the list to the food you suspect least. However, to make things more pleasant and varied, we suggest avoiding meat the first day. Then you could alternate meats, dairy foods or grains with fruits and vegetables.

You Eat Normally While Testing Foods

Each test meal should be normal-sized. Because each meal is composed of only a single food, you will probably require 3–4 times as much of that one food as you would normally eat when it is mixed with other foods. For instance, if you normally eat only a single potato with a meal, you may require 3–4 potatoes to make a full meal. Any snack you eat should also consist exclusively of the food being tested.

Eat each test meal within the same time that you normally take to consume a conventional plateful—20 minutes at most. And try to space your meals well apart. (Example: breakfast 7:30, lunch 12:30, dinner 7:30.)

Drugs May Confuse Test Results

Throughout the test period, except when testing a beverage, drink only pure water. Chewing gum is forbidden as are smoking, alcohol and drugs.

If you do smoke, drink alcohol or take a drug, it will invariably provoke a reaction and test out as allergenic. Should you be unable to complete the fast and test period without foregoing aspirin or a prescription drug, recognize that the drug will invoke a continual reaction. Any other allergenic reaction will be superimposed upon it. Knowing this, you may still be able to identify any flare-up caused by the allergenic foods you are testing. But drugs only confuse the task of identifying food allergens. If at all possible, you should drop all drugs in advance of commencing the fast.

A Simple Food Test Helps Roberta A.
End Her Arthritis

Roberta A. a 38-year old waitress, had had rheumatoid arthritis in her left knee for 18 months. Beside the routine 15 aspirin per day and occasional steroid injections, her doctor advised wearing a rubber stocking over her knee. But it didn't really help. After one particularly painful flare-up, Roberta had to give up her job. Unable to climb stairs any longer, she slept on the living room sofa. Even then, the pain was so severe she could sleep only when tranquilized.

A friend who worked in a health food store told Roberta about recent research that had identified food allergies as the cause of rheumatoid arthritis.

With her friend's help, Roberta reviewed her diet and found that each day she ate ten thick slices of whole wheat bread spread with peanut butter plus six cups of strong coffee plus eggs, beef, cheese and a large helping of spaghetti made from wheat. On Roberta's list of suspect foods were wheat, coffee, yeast, peanuts, eggs, beef and cheese.

Under her friend's direction, Roberta was to fast for 4 days after which she was to eat one suspect food each day for the following 7 days.

As she broke the fast on the fifth morning, Roberta realized that much of the pain had disappeared from her knee. But after her first two meals of cooked wheat, she was back on the sofa with one of the worst flare-ups she had ever experienced. Of the other foods, only coffee, beef and cheese precipitated arthritis symptoms.

Roberta dropped these four culprit foods and replaced them with health-building foods suggested by her friend. In 14 days, the pain and swelling in her knee had almost disappeared. A month later she was walking freely. In the 12 months since, she has worked steadily at her job. And only once, when she strayed from her diet, did her pains briefly return.

(*Note:* Four of Roberta's foods were Stressor Foods which we would not need to test.)

How Test Foods Should Be Prepared

Each food should be prepared the way you normally eat it either cooked or raw. If you eat it both ways, eat half the meal cooked, half raw. Buy foods from the same sources as usual. If you normally buy lettuce in the supermarket, don't get organically grown lettuce for the test. If you normally eat a certain grade of meat, test that grade not another grade that may have more or less fat. If you normally eat apples with the skins on, don't peel them for the test. You may be reacting to pesticide residues on the skin.

Foods such as honey, yeast or spices cannot form a regular

meal. Yet each must be tested singly like any other food and allotted the same period of time for any reaction to show up. Here is how certain foods should be tested.

BAKER'S YEAST: stir one tablespoon of commercial baker's yeast into a glass of pure, chlorine-free water and drink.

BREWER'S YEAST: stir one tablespoon of brewer's yeast into a glass of pure, chlorine-free water and drink.

OATS: half the meal should consist of plain, dry puffed oats and half of plain oatmeal prepared in pure, unchlorinated water.

RYE: boil some plain rye ears in a double cooker or over a slow burner. Use only pure, unchlorinated water. You may also add rye crackers made without yeast or sugar.

WHEAT: boil some plain wheat ears or cracked wheat in a double cooker or over a slow burner. Use only pure, unchlorinated water. Alternatively, make some chapattis (pancakes) of whole wheat flour and pure water. Sometimes matzoh is also made of pure wheat.

HONEY: stir 3 tablespoons of honey into a glass of warm, pure water and drink. Similar amounts of any other sweetener may be tested in the same manner.

SPICES, CONDIMENTS: pepper, MSG, vinegar, salt and similar spices or condiments must be tested by eating them on a food to which you know you are not allergic. Among foods least likely to be allergenic are cruciferous family vegetables (see Chapter 7) and deep ocean fish (not other seafood). Prepare a standard-sized meal composed exclusively of these foods and nothing else at all and season liberally with a single one of the condiments to be tested. Garlic and most herbs are not usually allergenic.

WATER: pure water, which includes most spring water, is never allergenic. But tap water treated with large amounts of chlorine, flouride, water-softening chemicals or other additives may very well be. Well water may also contain heavy pesticide or fertilizer residues. Mineral-rich spa water could also be allergenic. Reserve a full meal period for testing suspected water and drink as much as you comfortably can. You can drink it warm if you prefer.

Bear in mind that any food which you normally prepare by

mixing with a considerable volume of water, such as oatmeal or grits, may not itself be allergenic. Your allergy may be to the treated water.

At each test meal, eat *only* the food you are testing and absolutely nothing else. Don't add salt, butter, pepper or any kind of condiment or seasoning. If you are testing potatoes, your meal should consist only of baked, boiled or steamed potatoes. Never fry or use any method of preparation that would introduce another food.

CHAPTER 7

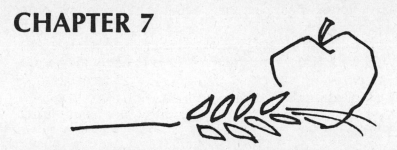

HOW TO IDENTIFY ALLERGY FOODS

After eating a test food, what reactions should you expect and when?

First, your test meals may reveal the existence of allergens that cause ailments other than arthritis, such as migraine headache. If this happens, you will naturally want to drop that food also even though it doesn't cause arthritis. Any food that produces dizziness, nausea, weakness, fatigue, fever or headache should be suspected as a possible cause of any other chronic ailment you might have. These symptoms can appear quite soon after eating the culprit food, sometimes within an hour.

Throughout your days of food testing, keep careful notes. Record the exact time of each meal and the times at which any symptoms appear.

Pinpointing the Foods That Cause Arthritis

How long does it take for symptoms to appear? After eating an arthritis-causing food, it usually takes 6–18 hours for arthritis symptoms and joint pains to appear. But during the first few days following the fast—when sensitivity is magnified—reactions may be even swifter. I have seen joint pains appear as rapidly as three hours after a test meal.

You will know which food causes any flare-up because, at latest, symptoms will appear first thing the following morning. Harking back to the sample test schedule in Chapter 6, if you woke up the first Wednesday with stiff and painful joints, you can be sure it was caused by the chicken you tested the previous day. (See page 96.)

Another example: Let's say that on the Saturday you experience a flare-up about 9 p.m. It had to be caused by the lamb you had been eating all day.

Again, if a flare-up occurred at noon on the second Tuesday while you were eating tomatoes, and continued at full strength for the remainder of the day while you continued with your tomato meals, the culprit food is almost certain to be tomatoes, the tomatoes you have been eating since breakfast.

There is, of course, a slight possibility it might have been caused by Monday night's soybean dinner, since you ate this dinner less than 18 hours previously. You would note down this overlapping possibility in your notebook.

A Simple Way to Identify Culprit Foods

Where there is any overlapping doubt as to exactly which of two foods may be causing arthritis, reading and writing tests can often help identify the non-tolerated food. Although reading and writing is affected only by the more severe allergens, these tests are often useful in confirming which of two or more suspect foods is the exact one to which you have a sensitivity.

Reading and writing tests must be made after each test meal. About thirty minutes after eating a test meal, begin to read a magazine. If the type appears blurred or you see double, this is a strong indication that the food you recently ate is allergenic.

For confirmation, write your name several times followed by a few sentences in longhand and two rows of figures. Then print a couple of sentences. If your writing tends to become a scrawl, or is barely legible, or if occasional letters or figures are omitted or written backwards, this is a strong indication that your last meal was allergenic.

These reading and writing checks must be made at intervals of 30 minutes for four hours following each test meal. If you get a reaction, the food may not necessarily be causing the arthritis. But you very probably have a strong sensitivity to it.

Reading and writing tests are now widely used in allergy

clinics to confirm food sensitivities. While testing foods for arthritis, they helped Myrtle L. uncover two migraine-causing food allergies that she would otherwise have overlooked completely.

Simple Food Tests Help Myrtle L. End the Pain of Both Arthritis and Migraine

For years, Myrtle L. a computer programmer, had been plagued with severe migraine attacks. Soon after her 39th birthday, pain and swelling appeared in Myrtle's wrists and soon spread to her elbows, knees and neck. After tests had confirmed that it was rheumatoid arthritis, a friend—who had already recovered from arthritis through nutritional therapy—suggested that Myrtle consult an allergist.

When the allergist discovered that Myrtle was a heavy eater of devitalized foods, he placed her on a five day fast. Most of her joint pains disappeared during the five foodless days. Myrtle then began to test a suspected Allergy Food at the rate of one per day.

At intervals of 30 minutes after each meal, she was instructed to read a magazine and to write several sentences in longhand and print. An hour after eating a plateful of cooked wheat, Myrtle could hardly read the magazine—the print was so blurred. And her usual firm, round handwriting became a barely legible scrawl. Several hours later, she experienced severe pain in her wrists and knees.

Myrtle noticed the same blurred vision and scrawled handwriting after meals of cheese and chocolate. But only the cheese produced arthritis pains. On the day following the chocolate tests, she experienced a severe attack of migraine headache.

After dropping all three foods, Myrtle's arthritis symptoms gradually disappeared. And her migraine attacks became increasingly rare.

How to Use the Same Techniques That Successful Arthritis Clinics Employ

The fasting and food testing methods described here are virtually identical with those being used in the most successful and most expensive allergy clinics that reverse thousands of cases of rheumatoid arthritis every year. By following instructions carefully, you can achieve the same results in your own home without spending a penny.

If, after a flare-up occurs, pain and stiffness have not decreased by at least 50 per cent, postpone testing the next food.

In its place enjoy a meal of deep ocean fish such as cod or haddock with cruciferous-family vegetables like cabbage, Brussels sprouts or broccoli. These are rarely allergenic. Then you can add a desert of gourd-family foods like melons, plus an avocado. Food families are listed later in this chapter. You may also add any food that you have already confirmed as a non-allergen.

How to Interpret Signs of Food Sensitivity

During food tests, flare-up symptoms usually begin to die down in a few hours after you stop eating the culprit food. Usually, pain and stiffness caused by a previous day's flare-up will decrease overnight.

However, before continuing with your tests, wait for symptoms to diminish to where you can readily recognize another flare-up if it occurs. Meanwhile, go on eating meals of fish with cruciferous and gourd family foods and avocadoes.

Usually you will not have to wait more than 24 hours before symptoms have abated to where you can continue testing. Continue to drink only pure water and add nothing at all to any meal but the foods just mentioned (no frying, butter or seasoning of any kind). As soon as symptoms have diminished appreciably, proceed with food testing.

Should you experience one or two prolonged flare-ups, you may not have sufficient time to test all ten suspect foods in the ten days at your disposal. In this event, you can test the remainder with the alternative techniques described in Chapter 8.

Provided you test foods in approximately the order you suspect them, two or three flare-ups should serve to identify the most potent allergens that are causing your arthritic disease.

Food Testing Helps Bob W. Phase Out Rheumatoid Arthritis

Forty-eight year old Bob W. had had rheumatoid arthritis for 3 years. His doctor prescribed drugs that suppressed the pain and swelling. But the side effects caused constant discomfort. Finally, Bob consulted a new doctor, a Holistically oriented physician well versed in nutrition. Bob was told to drop all Stressor Foods. Despite this, Bob continued to experience bouts of intense pain in his knees and wrists.

His doctor sent Bob to a small arthritis clinic in the Southwest for fasting and food testing. Bob was delighted when, after five days of fasting, his pains disappeared. He then began to test 9 suspected foods—one each day. Beginning 30 minutes after each meal, Bob was instructed to give himself a reading and handwriting test.

The first flare-up occurred just after noon on the second day. The nutritionist-in-charge could not be absolutely certain whether it was caused by the day's breakfast or by the previous night's dinner. For both meals had been eaten within 18 overlapping hours of the flare-up.

A quick look at Bob's reading and writing records confirmed that Bob had experienced blurred vision that had begun about an hour after breakfast that morning and Bob's handwriting had become noticeably shaky and unreadable. On this basis, the nutritionist decided it was the breakfast food that had triggered the arthritis.

Two other flare-ups that followed occurred on rising and were clearly associated with the previous day's food.

Altogether, Bob tested allergy-positive to wheat, rice and corn. These foods were dropped immediately.

A week later, the pain and swelling in Bob's joints had subsided once more. He strictly followed his dietary instructions and he has been free of arthritis for more than a year.

An Easy Way to Trace Arthritis-Causing Food Families

Most people with arthritic disease find they are allergic to several foods, not just one. Some people have shown allergy reactions to as many as 15 or more different foods.

In many cases, people with multiple sensitivities react to several closely related foods that allergists group together in a single family. The food families are related in that all members of one family are recognized by the immune system as having the same "foreign" antigen.

For example, two fairly common arthritis-causing allergens, potatoes and tomatoes, both belong to the nightshade family. Many people who are sensitive to tomatoes are also sensitive to potatoes, and vice versa. These people have a predisposed sensitivity towards other members of the nightshade family such as green and red peppers, eggplant and paprika.

If tests confirm that you are allergic to any food belonging to a common food family, you may well have a cross-sensitivity to other foods in the same family. This knowledge is extremely helpful in tracking down arthritis-causing allergens.

For instance, a normal meal might contain both a potato and a tomato. Together, these two are sufficient to induce an arthritic flare-up. But if you omitted either the potato or the tomato, the remaining food may not be sufficient to produce a rejection response by the immune system. This is why we eat a full-sized meal of each suspected food during a test.

Here are the principal food families. Not all are common allergens. The cruciferous and gourd families are rarely allergenic.

Common Food Family Groups

ASTER: artichoke, camomile, dandelion, endive, escarole, goldenrod, lettuce, safflower oil, sunflower oil, sunflower seeds.

BOVINE: beef, goat, lamb, mutton, veal. All milk and dairy products.

CITRUS: all citrus fruits.

CRUCIFEROUS: broccoli, Brussels sprouts, cabbage, cauliflower, Chinese celery, collards, horseradish, kale, kohlrabi, mustard, mustard greens, radish, rutabagas, turnip.

GRASS: all cereal grains including bamboo shoots, barley, corn, malt, millet, molasses, oats, rice, rye, sorghum and wheat. Also sprouts of any of these grains.

GOURD: cantaloupe, cucumber, melons—all types— pumpkin, squash, watermelon, zucchini. Also seeds of these plants.

LEGUMES: alfalfa, mung beans, peanuts, soybean and soy products, all beans and peas, lecithin and licorice. Also pea, bean and alfalfa sprouts.

NIGHTSHADE: cayenne pepper, chili pepper, green and red peppers, eggplant, paprika, potato and tomato.

PARSLEY: anise, carrot, celeriac, celery, chervil, coriander, cumin, dill, fennel, parsnip. Also seeds of these plants.

PLUM: almond, apricot, cherry, nectarine, peach, persimmon, plum, prune, wild cherry.

ROSE: blackberry, boysenberry, dewberry, loganberry, raspberry, rose hip, strawberry, youngberry.

YEAST: baker's and brewer's yeast.

The Worst Arthritis-Causing Food

Population studies show that arthritis is most common in countries where wheat is the staple food. Wheat is possibly the most common arthritis-causing allergen. Scientists have discovered that many people, including some who have never had arthritis before, can produce arthritis symptoms in a relatively short time when an extract of wheat is placed under the tongue.

Investigation has shown that sensitivity is usually to gluten, a protein found in wheat and also in all other cereals. Hence if you show a confirmed sensitivity to wheat or to any other grains, you should suspect all other members of the grass family.

Wheat products, which may provoke the same sensitivity as wheat itself, are found in a wide variety of processed foods such as bread, baked goods, beer, liquor, mayonnaise, pasta, ice cream and most sausages. Corn products are also common ingredients in processed foods. Many alcoholic drinks contain large amounts of various grains as well as sugar and yeast.

Other Common Foods That Cause Arthritis

The same can be said of soybean and soy products. Processed foods may contain varying amounts of many basic foods, each of which could be allergenic. Which is one reason why you should stay strictly away from *all* processed foods from now on.

The nightshade family is another group of fairly common arthritis-causing allergens. Besides provoking an immune response, these foods contain solanine, a glyco-alkaloid which inhibits the action of cholinasterase, the enzyme that provides flexibility and agility in muscles.

Although brewer's yeast is recognized as a splendid source of B-complex vitamins, it is also a protein-rich micro-organism. Tiny particles of this protein may be recognized as a foreign antigen in the bloodstream. The same is true of baker's yeast used in making most (but not all) breads.

Protein-rich foods like cereal gluten, meats, eggs, chicken, yeast, soybeans and dairy foods are by far the most common arthritis-causing allergens. With minor exceptions, the less protein a food contains, the less likely it is to be recognized as a foreign antigen when entering the bloodstream.

The safest form of whole protein is a low-fat ocean fish like cod or haddock.

Audrey M's Food Sleuthing Pays Off by Eliminating Her Arthritis

Audrey M. a 45-year old nurse, had had rheumatoid arthritis for several years. Through reading medical journals she had become aware of the growing scientific evidence that food allergies are the most probable cause of rheumatoid arthritis.

Audrey didn't have time to fast but felt certain she was addicted to what she called her "arthritis trigger," a hefty sandwich of lettuce, Swiss cheese and tomato placed between two slices of whole wheat bread generously spread with peanut butter.

Audrey knew that, except for the fat in the cheese, these were all considered healthful foods. Yet each was also a fairly common arthritis allergen. Moreover one of the sandwiches formed the core of every meal and snack that Audrey ate. Each day, she ate at least six large sandwiches and often seven or eight.

If a meal or snack didn't include her favorite sandwich, Audrey felt quite uncomfortable. The discomfort would increase until she was able to eat the addictive food once more.

Helping to confirm her suspicions was the fact that Audrey felt stuffed and gassy soon after eating a sandwich and she experienced frequent diarrhea. After one particularly painful flare-up, Audrey psyched herself up to eliminate the "arthritis trigger."

Once Audrey actually stopped eating the sandwich, benefits soon began to appear. Within three days, her digestive problems had cleared up completely. And the pain and swelling in her wrists and knees grew noticeably less.

But a continuous low-level pain lingered on. Audrey knew enough of nutrition to realize it was probably because she was still eating some of the ingredients found in the bread; or because she was still eating a food of the same family as those in her sandwich.

Right away, Audrey cut out all other foods containing wheat or yeast together with sour cream, potatoes, corn and soybeans—foods she regularly ate that belonged to the same families as the foods in her sandwich.

A week after dropping all these foods, the last of Audrey's arthritis pain and inflammation disappeared. Later, when she underwent a fast and food testing, Audrey found she was sensitive to only half the foods she had eliminated. She discovered she could safely go on eating tomatoes, potatoes, peanuts and soybeans.

But as a temporary expedient, her makeshift sleuthing had proved remarkably successful.

Purging Arthritis or Gout by Eliminating Destructive Foods

By now, you should have identified all of the allergenic foods that are causing your arthritic disease. Or if any doubt exists as to which of two overlapping foods are allergenic, you can test each one again by the alternative tests described in Chapter 8. Likewise, if you were unable to test all the foods on your list, you can test the remainder the same way.

In any case, by eliminating *all* of these foods from your diet—including those you have not yet tested or confirmed— you should be well on the way towards ending the pain, stiffness and inflammation arising from rheumatoid and similar forms of arthritic disease caused by auto-immunity. As osteoarthritis and gout pain may also be worsened by auto-immunity, eliminating the responsible allergenic foods may significantly help to reduce pain from these diseases also.

To completely overcome gout, you must cut out all Stressor Foods together with the special gout-aggravating foods listed in

Chapter 10, and you must bring your weight back down to normal.

To completely overcome osteo-arthritis, you must cut out all the Stressor Foods described in Chapter 10 and bring your weight down to normal.

How Other Food Testing Methods Can Help

What if you completely overlooked an allergenic food while compiling your list of suspected foods? The food would not have been tested and you might still be eating it every day. As a result, arthritis pain would still be with you.

If you have any type of arthritis other than gout or osteo-arthritis and if pain, stiffness and inflammation have continued after the fast and through the food-testing period, this may be the explanation.

You can easily test any suspect foods you may have overlooked by using the alternative techniques described in the next chapter.

Meanwhile, once your tests are over and you have eliminated both Stressor and Allergenic Foods from your diet, you can go ahead and combine any number of compatible foods to form any meal that you desire.

CHAPTER 8

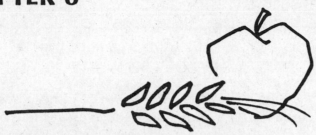

HOW TO SELF-TEST YOUR OWN ALLERGIES TO ARTHRITIS-CAUSING FOODS

Elizabeth D. was one of hundreds of arthritis sufferers I met who had retired to the Southwest in the hope of finding relief through the dry climate. Elizabeth did eventually find relief, though not through low humidity.

"I first had pain and swelling in my hands, then it spread to my elbows, shoulders and knees," she told me. "My doctor diagnosed it as rheumatoid arthritis. He placed me on fifteen aspirin a day. That didn't help, so he gave me Indocin and later a steroid. They helped briefly but only in large doses.

"At forty-seven I could barely walk a block without crippling pain. I'd lost twenty-five pounds and I was as thin as a rake. So my husband retired here after thirty years in the service. We thought the climate might help. But that was another disappointment.

"Then I got pneumonia. Our new family physician here said it was because the steroid I was taking suppressed my immune system so much that I had no resistance. I also found that the steroid was causing bone loss. And the fifteen daily aspirin were causing severe gastritis and ringing in my ears.

"The drugs had me really scared! Not far away is an arthritis clinic. They use fasting to find out which foods cause arthritis. I didn't really believe in it all. But I was so desperate I got my husband to drive me there. They said I was too thin to fast, but they did have an alternative method.

"They used a pulse test that somebody developed back in the nineteen-thirties. Whenever you eat a food that you're sensitive to, your pulse rate rises. Of couse, you have to stop taking medication. The whole thing was so simple I could have done it myself at home. Anyway, they found I was allergic to beef, eggs, milk, chocolate, pork and luncheon meats.

"Of course, they didn't know which of these was actually causing arthritis. So they told me to cut all of them out of my diet. They also gave me a list of high-risk foods to avoid and another list of natural foods I should eat instead.

"Well, I never really believed it would work, but I followed their advice anyway. Believe it or not, after a month on this food, the pain and swelling in my joints started to die down. After three months, I could walk a mile without pain. My weight gradually came back up to normal.

"The only flare-up I've had was when we went to a dude ranch for a week and I went on a beef kick. I swear I'll never do anything like it again. It undid the work of months. This time, I'm sticking right to my diet. Besides, it helps me stay completely regular. I'm fifty-two now. I'm completely free of arthritis and I feel twice as good as I ever did before."

All Allergy Foods Should Be Eliminated

Elizabeth's recovery is typical of many I encountered where, for one reason or another, a fast could not be used. If you are underweight or unable to fast, or if you cannot spare the time, there *are* alternatives. The alternative food tests don't necessarily tell you exactly which foods are causing arthritis. But they can identify most foods to which you may be sensitive.

Whether or not a food sensitivity is causing arthritis, it's wise to cut it out anyway.

Before we go on, I'd like to emphasize this. Don't be tempted to by-pass the fasting test and use one or other of the alternative tests because they sound easier. They are second choice alternatives, not substitutes.

None will stop rheumatoid arthritis pain in its tracks like a fast. Nor do they magnify test reactions to reveal low level food allergies that may be causing arthritis.

How Your Pulse Can Reveal Hidden Food Allergies

The best alternative test for food sensitivity is the Pulse Test. This method was first developed in the 1930s by Dr. Arthur Coca, a famous immunologist. When his wife became ill, Dr. Coca discovered that she became worse after eating specific foods which increased her pulse rate. When these foods were eliminated, his wife recovered.

Other allergists have refined and improved the method since. But the technique is still basically the one developed by Dr. Coca. Together with fasting, it has almost completely replaced such traditional methods as skin-testing for food allergies. And the wonderful thing about it is that you can do it yourself at home with results as good as those obtained by any professional allergist.

Before you can use the Pulse Test, you must first establish your normal pulse rate and your normal pulse limits. To do so, you take your pulse 14 times a day for 3 consecutive days immediately prior to testing the foods.

As a preliminary, practice feeling your pulse a few times with the tip of your thumb. Your pulse is located in the underside of your forearm about an inch above the wrist on the thumb side. Practice taking your pulse several times for 30 seconds while you time yourself with the sweep hand of a watch or clock or with a digital timepiece that shows seconds. If you count 35 beats in 30 seconds, your pulse rate is 70 beats per minute.

Finding Your Normal Pulse Rate

To establish your normal pulse rate you must read your pulse for 3 consecutive days immediately prior to food testing like this:

1. Immediately on waking and while still lying in bed.
2. Immediately prior to each meal.

3. At 30, 60 and 90 minutes after each meal.

4. Immediately before retiring.

Except when taking your pulse in bed as you awaken, take all the other readings while seated. Note down the time and number of beats for each reading in a notebook.

Here is an example:

	Day 1	Day 2	Day 3
On rising	60	59	59
Before breakfast	58	57	60
30 minutes after breakfast	68	67	68
60 minutes after breakfast	74	70	74
90 minutes after breakfast	70	66	70
Before lunch	63	62	66
30 minutes after lunch	74	71	74
60 minutes after lunch	76	72	77
90 minutes after lunch	70	67	75
Before dinner	68	62	65
30 minutes after dinner	77	68	76
60 minutes after dinner	75	70	79
90 minutes after dinner	73	67	77
On retiring	70	63	70
Daily totals	976	921	990
	÷14	÷14	÷14
Average daily rate	69.7	65.7	70.7
Normal pulse rate	69		
Daily high	77	72	79
Daily low	58	57	59
Differential	19	15	20
Normal high rate	76		

To find your daily average rate, total the 14 daily readings and divide by 14.

To find your normal daily pulse rate, total the average daily pulse rates for each of the 3 days and divide by 3. (Example: 69.7 + 65.7 + 70.7 = 206.1 ÷ 3 = 68.7 which we round off to 69.)

To find your daily differential, subtract the lowest reading of each day from the highest reading of each day. (Example for Day 1: 77 − 58 = 19.)

To find your normal high rate, total the three daily high rates and divide by 3. (Example: $77 + 72 + 79 = 228 \div 3 = 76$.)

Your Pulse Indicates Your Inner Health

Now examine the pulse readings in your notebook for each of the 3 days.

If on any day, the differential between the highest and lowest readings exceeds 12, it probably indicates sensitivity to a food that you ate that day. If this differential on any day is below 12, no food sensitivity is indicated.

If the average daily high reading varies from day to day by more than 2, it again indicates a probable food sensitivity. If the daily high rate remains constant, it probably means you are not sensitive to any foods you ate during the 3-day period.

In our sample pulse observations, two readings indicate the probability of one or more food sensitivities. For example, on all 3 days, a differential of more than 12 indicates a strong probability that at least one allergenic food was eaten on all 3 days.

Again, the variation in the daily high rate exceeds 12, again indicating the probable existence of a food sensitivity.

If your notes show that your pulse rose to more than six beats per minute over and above your normal pulse rate after eating any particular food, test those foods first.

In your notebook you must also record the basic food contents of all foods you eat at each meal, including any beverages. Snacks, beverages or chewing gum should not be taken between meals as they may distort pulse readings.

Preparing for the Pulse Test

Take your pulse only after you have been seated for several minutes. If you find a high reading, be sure it is not due to exercise, emotional stress, excitement, an infection or infectious disease or severe sunburn. Any sudden increase *not* due to one of these causes is probably due to a sensitivity to a food or to an environmental allergy.

You can usually detect a sensitivity due to something in the environment such as dust, pollen, animal danders or chemicals because your pulse will remain high the entire time you remain in that environment. If this happens, try changing your environment while you continue to eat the same foods. If you had an environmental allergy, your pulse rate should gradually drop back to normal. If your pulse rate remains high, it could mean you are allergic to one or more of the foods you are eating.

All prerequisites that applied to food testing after a fast apply equally to pulse testing. You must first make a list of suspect foods to be tested (Chapter 6) and you should avoid testing Stressor Foods. Only basic foods should be tested.

All smoking and medication should be stopped at least 3 days prior to establishing your normal pulse rate and they must be withheld throughout the food tests that follow. Any food to be tested must have been eaten regularly and at least once during the 5 days preceding the pulse tests.

If while establishing your normal pulse rate, your notes show that your pulse rose to more than six beats over and above your normal pulse rate after eating any particular foods, test those foods first.

All foods to be tested should be prepared as described in Chapter 6 for the fasting test. As after fasting, you test only one food at a time. But with the pulse test you can test as many as 3 foods in one day—one at a time, of course.

Mini-Meals Give Best Results

Prepare the same normal-sized meal of the food to be tested, exactly as for the fasting method. But—and here's the difference. For pulse testing, divide that meal into 3 equal portions. And eat each portion 60 minutes apart.

There's one important rule to observe: if immediately prior to the time when you should eat the next mini-meal, your pulse is reading above its normal daily rate, postpone eating until it drops to normal or below and has stayed in that range for a full hour.

Suppose you were testing wheat, beef and oatmeal. Assuming it takes ten minutes to eat a mini-meal, your eating schedule might look like this:

7:30 a.m.	Wheat
8:40 a.m.	Wheat
9:50 a.m.	Wheat
12:30 p.m.	Beef

1:40 p.m.	Beef
2:50 p.m.	Beef
6:30 p.m.	Oats
7:40 p.m.	Oats
8:50 p.m.	Oats

You would eat at these times only if your pulse reads normal or below. The advantage of eating small mini-meals is that the amount of food is not sufficiently large to cause any significant increase in heart rate due to the added task of digestion. At all times, only pure water should be drunk. Any suspected beverage must be tested as though it were a food as described in Chapter 6.

If your pulse is above normal at any time you are scheduled to begin another mini-meal, wait for it to drop to normal. Then allow it to beat for one full hour at the normal rate or lower before you eat.

Now for the actual food testing.

What Your Pulse Tells About the Foods You Eat

Go ahead and eat your first mini-meal.

Immediately after eating, take your pulse and record it, together with a notation of the time and the food you are testing, in your notebook.

Do the same thing 30 minutes later.

Now, compare your pulse rate immediately after eating with the rate 30 minutes later.

If it has increased by 15 beats per minute or more, this indicates a strong probability that you are sensitive to the test food.

If at the 30 minute reading, your pulse reads six beats or more per minute above your normal high rate, this again indicates a strong possibility of sensitivity to the test food.

If both events occur together, you can regard this as an almost certain indication of a strong sensitivity.

Again, if 30 minutes after the test meal your pulse reads 84 beats per minute or higher, this is another almost certain indication that you have eaten an allergenic food.

When interpreting these results, be sure of course that you

are free of any emotional stress, excitement, infection, heavy sunburn or the effects of recent exercise.

Repeat this process with each mini-meal of the day.

For each test food, compare results for each of the 3 mini-meals. If any sensitivity indications were repeated 2 or 3 times, this is almost certain proof that your immune system has a strong rejectivity response to that food.

That food should be dropped from your diet, at least until you have a chance to confirm the sensitivity by fasting or other methods.

Provided you have eaten the test food regularly right up to the date your food testing begins, you can continue testing suspect foods for five more full days. Just to make this clear, you can continue to eat suspect foods freely during the 3 days you are establishing your normal pulse rate. The 5 days we're talking about begin with your first day of actual food testing.

On this basis and assuming no delays, you should be able to test 15 different foods during the 5 test days.

A Simple Diet Change Brings Speedy Relief to Doreen P's Pain-Crippled Knee

Can alternative tests actually help get rid of arthritis?

"The pain was like a sword driven through my knee," this is a 54-year old woman speaking.

"It was so bad I could not place any weight on my left knee at all. I had to give up driving and stay at home."

Can you imagine such excruciating agony? But that was 3 years ago. The lady now is a picture of glowing good health. Standing beside the swimming pool at a large Arizona adult community, Doreen P. had just swum a mile non-stop.

"But three years ago, I was crippled by rheumatoid arthritis. My physician started me off with fourteen aspirin a day. Then he tried cortisone. But the side effects were so disturbing I had to go back to aspirin.

"We'd heard about fasting and elimination diets. But the arthritis left me completely emaciated. Fasting was out of the question.

"Then a friend told us about a naturopath who was getting good results with arthritis without fasting. My husband drove me to see him. In one long afternoon session he taught us the basics of sound nutrition. Then he taught us how to use the pulse test and the kinesiology method for testing food.

"We did the tests ourselves at home. The pulse test showed that I was allergy-positive to sugar, milk, beef, chicken, chocolate and coffee—favorite foods that I'd eaten all my life. The kinesiology tests confirmed the results.

"I hated to give up those foods I loved. But four weeks later I was walking without pain. You couldn't have got me to eat any of those foods again for a million dollars.

"Eventually, by trial and error we found that only the sugar, milk, chocolate and coffee were causing arthritis. The beef and chicken didn't seem to be causing anything in particular. So I just eat them occasionally, once in a while.

"Right after that my husband retired. We moved here and I haven't had a touch of arthritis since."

A Quick Method for Testing Any Food

At any time when you have met the requirements for food testing, you can use this Quick Pulse Test to check out any food in under an hour. You can do so without having to establish your normal pulse rate in advance.

The requirements are that you must have eaten the test food at least once within the previous 5 days. You must not have smoked or taken any drugs within 3 days or any stimulant such as alcohol or coffee for at least 24 hours. You must feel free of emotional stress, excitement, infection, heavy sunburn or the effects of exercise. And you must be free of the effects of any environmental allergy.

You will get a stronger reaction if you last ate the test food exactly 5 days previously and have not eaten it since.

The test must be made on an empty stomach. Hence it is best made at breakfast time.

Begin by taking your pulse a few minutes after rising. Take it while seated.

Then eat a light meal of the test food. The amount to eat is about half the size of a regular breakfast. Eat nothing but the test food and drink nothing but pure water.

After eating, wait 30 minutes and take your pulse. If after eating your pulse has risen by 15–20 beats per minute over the reading you got before the meal, this is a good indication of a sensitivity to that food.

Provided the requirements are always met, you can repeat this test once at breakfast time on any day. The test is quite reliable and can serve to confirm previous tests.

You can also use this test to prove to yourself that drugs or stimulants always test allergy-positive. After taking medication or smoking a cigarette or drinking two cups of strong coffee or two alcoholic drinks, your pulse will almost always show a strong sensitivity reaction within 10–30 minutes.

The Quick Pulse Test Helps John L. Identify the Cause of His Arthritis

The Quick Pulse Test is essentially the same technique that helped John L. locate the cause of his arthritis.

"I'd *been* to an arthritis clinic. I'd *learned* all about fasting, nutrition and natural foods. I'd *changed* my diet completely. But I *still* had rheumatoid arthritis."

John L., a former Navy officer who had been forced to retire because of arthritis, tells this story.

"They'd told me at the clinic that I shouldn't smoke or drink beer. Of course, everyone knows that smoking is bad for health. But I just couldn't see how smoking or alcohol could affect arthritis."

John described how he found a book on pulse testing for food allergies written years ago.

"All you had to do was to eat a meal of just one food and take your pulse thirty minutes later. Well, one day I noticed that after a cigarette my pulse rate rose eighteen beats a minute. After two cans of beer it rose twenty-two beats a minute. According to the book, these were danger signals.

"It scared the daylights out of me! I quit smoking and drinking right there, cold turkey! Three weeks later, my arthritis had faded away.

"I did have three flare-ups afterwards. But the last was five years ago. I've stuck with the diet and I've steered clear of cigarettes and beer and I've been totally free of arthritis ever since."

How to Tap in to Your Body's Instinctual Wisdom

There's an even swifter method for testing for food sensitivity. It is so incredibly simple that, frankly, I didn't believe it until I saw it actually demonstrated and yielding accurate results.

It's based on a natural therapy called kinesiology which works on the principal that the body itself knows what may be wrong with it and what needs to be done to restore health.

Now that's not so far-fetched. When animals get sick, they listen to their instinctual body wisdom which tells them to stop eating and to fast. Fasting frees the body from the task of digestion and permits self-healing to proceed at the fastest possible rate.

Studies have also shown that if given the choice of a wide variety of basic foods (no sugar, sweets, ice cream or other junk food) both animals and children will automatically select those foods containing the nutritional elements that their body needs most.

To use kinesiology, we must learn to read the signals our body is giving us. When we feed our body a food which our immune system rejects, the body will let us know right away that this sensitivity exists.

How to Put Test Foods into Your Bloodstream in Seconds

The simplest way to learn how well the body tolerates any particular food is by observing a reflex that exists between tongue, immune system and brain. The effect of this reflex is to reduce the strength of muscles throughout the body.

This phenomenon has long been known to medical science. It is extensively used every day by tens of millions of heart disease patients all over the U.S. and throughout the world to relieve angina attacks.

An angina attack is an unbearable pain in the chest that foreshadows a heart attack. People with heart disease suffer frequently from these pains. Any angina attack can develop into a heart attack. To prevent a heart attack, doctors prescribe nitroglycerine tablets to be taken at the first sign of angina pain. The nitroglycerine relaxes blood vessels and prevents the blockage of a coronary artery that would otherwise precipitate a heart attack.

When an angina pain occurs, a heart attack may follow in just two or three minutes. Somehow, that nitroglycerine has to be placed in the bloodstream in mere seconds. The pain of angina is such that a victim could not possibly inject the nitroglycerine himself. And if simply swallowed, it would take 10–15 minutes to enter the bloodstream.

Instead, at the first hint of angina pain, a nitroglycerine tablet is placed *under the tongue.* Here it is immediately absorbed into the bloodstream, and within seconds it reaches the coronary arteries.

Not only nitroglycerine but *any* food placed under the tongue is absorbed into the body immediately. It is through this same access that tiny particles of undigested food enter the bloodstream and provoke a rejectivity response. Other more numerous particles are absorbed later through the intestines.

A Simple Kinesiology Technique That Identifies Disease-Causing Foods

When the immune system rejects particles of a non-tolerated food, a neurological reflex relays this information to the brain. The brain reacts by reducing the strength and power in our body muscles. The entire process works about as swiftly, and in somewhat the same way, as the knee jerk reflex.

Within 30 seconds of placing a sample of test food under the tongue, we start to lose an appreciable degree of muscular strength.

This is how kinesiology food testing works! By placing a sample of the test food under the tongue, a person's sensitivity to that food can be detected by simply measuring muscle strength 30–90 seconds later.

The same requirements are necessary for kinesiological testing as for pulse or fasting tests. No smoking or drugs during the preceding 3 days and no coffee or alcohol within 24 hours. Any food to be tested should have been eaten fairly regularly and at least once during the preceding 5 days. And you should be emotionally calm, relaxed and feeling well.

The tests should be made on a relatively empty stomach.

Thus we suggest doing any kinesiological testing before eating the first meal of the day.

Reading Your Body's Danger Signals

To conduct a test, you need a second person.

Begin by holding out your arm horizontally to the side, palm down. Keep the arm firm, straight and rigid.

The other person then grasps your wrist with one hand and presses firmly and steadily downwards until your arm is forced down to your side. It must be done smoothly and without jerking. The person gauges the strength required to overcome your resistance.

Next, lower your arm and chew a small piece of test food. Masticate it and mix it well with saliva. Then place it under your tongue and keep it there until the test is over. Let exactly 60 seconds tick away on your watch.

Then hold your arm out again and have the person press it down to your side. If your resistance weakens appreciably, this indicates a food sensitivity. If your muscle strength remains constant, the food is unlikely to be allergenic.

Immediately when the test is over, rinse the food out of your mouth. Don't swallow it.

If you got no reaction you can continue testing with another food. If the food tested allergy-positive, sit down and rest for ten minutes before testing the next food.

At any one session you can test half a dozen different foods. To test a liquid, take a mouthful, work it around your mouth for 15 seconds until well mixed with saliva, then hold it under the tongue as if it were a food. Any beverages should be prepared double strength.

As with all other food testing methods, keep detailed notes of all test results together with dates and times. If you detect any sensitivities, you can recheck them again later or the following day for confirmation.

Claudia A. Lets Her Body's Own Wisdom Guide Her to Freedom from Arthritis

When I first saw kinesiology food testing demonstrated, I could hardly wait to try it out on someone with arthritis. My opportunity came just days later.

Three years earlier Claudia A. had hit her right knee on a desk. Arthritis pains soon began. Within months, pain and inflammation spread to the fingers and wrist of her right hand. Her doctor prescribed large doses of aspirin, but her joints still felt as though they were on fire, and every morning her hand and leg were painfully stiff.

Claudia jumped at the chance to try kinesiology and food elimination. She made a list of foods she craved most. To let the stiffness work out of her joints, we did the testing in mid-afternoon. Claudia skipped breakfast and lunch and took the tests on an empty stomach.

Claudia didn't have much muscle strength left. But I detected a distinct weakening after she took mouthfuls of sugar, wheat, egg and cheese.

I advised Claudia to try cutting out these foods along with several other health-robbing Stressor Foods. And, of course, to stay off aspirin.

A month later, a cheerful Claudia phoned to say her arthritis was much improved. She could move her knee and hand without pain, but there were heavy cracking noises.

That sounded like calcium deposits. I told Claudia to keep moving her joints gently to help the calcium break up. I also suggested eating natural foods rich in calcium.

Three months later a letter arrived from a joyous Claudia. She had written to show how well she could now use her formerly crippled hand. Claudia was walking again and doing housework and had totally recovered.

A Slow but Often Sure Way to Eliminate Arthritis Pain

The Food Elimination Test is yet another, albeit much slower method of food testing for allergies.

There are two requirements. First you must prepare a list of suspect foods as described in Chapter 6.

Second, you must cut out all Stressor Foods at least 3 days prior to beginning the test, and you must eliminate them permanently. As you'll recall after reading Chapter 9, Stressor Foods include smoking, drugs, alcohol and caffeine. All four always test allergy-positive, and all are prime causes of arthritis and gout as well as other life-threatening diseases.

The only possible exception would be to continue with a prescription drug which is essential for the preservation of life. And you should ask your doctor for his permission to phase this out as you improve.

If you cannot possibly go on without aspirin or other pain-relieving drugs, then try to reduce the dosage to the bare minimum. Until all medication is stopped, you are likely to always have some arthritic pain. But you should not stop taking any medication essential to life without your doctor's approval.

The Broadside Approach to Nutritional Therapy

The test simply consists of eliminating all of the foods on your suspect list together with any other foods belonging to the same families. For example, if wheat is one of the foods to be eliminated, the entire grass family must also be cut out including corn and oats. (Food families are listed in Chapter 7.)

All of the foods must be eliminated simultaneousiy at the start of the test. Since you will cut out all of the foods that you crave and eat most of, you will probably experience noticeable withdrawal symptoms during the first few days.

Since there is no fast to speed up the disappearance of rheumatoid arthritis pain, arthritis symptoms will be slower to clear up. Expect ten days to elapse before any noticeable improvement.

Then if you have eliminated all of the foods to which you are sensitive, arthritis pain and inflammation should begin to show steady improvement.

Although this method can be quite successful, the chances are that you will have cut out many foods to which you are not actually sensitive.

Assuming that arthritis symptoms disappear, you can usually identify specific allergen foods by introducing one food at a time back into your diet.

The Way to Confirm a Suspected Allergen

Let's say you introduce corn back into your diet. Do so for a period of 12 days. If no symptoms of arthritis or other disease appear, then introduce a second food for a period of 12 days. As soon as symptoms appear, drop the food you have just introduced. If symptoms gradually disappear you will know that food is allergenic.

With patience, you can work through your entire list of suspect foods and confirm which actually cause arthritis symptoms and which do not. The method is necessarily slow because you lose sensitivity to foods after you have eliminated them from your diet for a period of weeks. It may take a few days for the sensitivity to reappear.

The advantage of the Food Elimination Test is that it doesn't need to interrupt your lifestyle or take up much time. Also it actually identifies specific foods that cause arthritic disease.

English Study Proves Allergy Foods Cause Rheumatoid Arthritis

An example of how the elimination diet works in practice was reported in *Clinical Allergy* (vol. 10, no. 4, 1980) in which 22 rheumatoid arthritis patients in England were placed on a diet that excluded all foods that are commonly allergenic.

The first sign of improvement began ten days after commencing the diet, and by the time the test was over, 20 of the 22 patients had found their arthritis symptoms relieved. Food tests then revealed that 14 of the patients had sensitivities to grains while whole milk, cheese, beef, eggs, chicken, liver and potatoes were other foods high on the list. When they tried eating these allergenic foods later, 19 of the patients found their arthritis symptoms had come back—in one case only two hours after eating.

Llewellyn R. Conquers Arthritis with the Food Elimination Test

Llewellyn R. stumbled on to the Food Elimination Test on his own.

"I read a Nature Cure book that listed about thirty different foods believed to cause arthritis," he told me.

"The pain and swelling in my joints was driving me crazy. I was so desperate I decided to just go ahead and cut out all thirty foods.

"Well, nothing happened for about a month. Then I noticed

my joint pains seemed less intense. I began to get periods of relief from pain—something I hadn't experienced for a year. In another few weeks, the pains had subsided almost entirely.

"Every week I felt better. The stiffness and inflammation disappeared. The book warned that calcium deposits would take time to break up and be absorbed. It recommended eating lots of green, leafy vegetables rich in calcium.

"What I ended up eating was practically nothing but fresh, raw salads of fruits and vegetables along with nuts, seeds, avocadoes and fish. Well, they did the trick. I recovered completely.

"The book didn't say I could eat any of the foods again. But I thought it unlikely that all thirty foods would be causing arthritis. So I started adding back one food every two weeks. If after two weeks nothing happened, I'd add another.

"A week after I started back on bread, I got a real swift flare-up. So bread was out for good.

"It took a year to test all thirty foods. But I found I could eat most of the foods quite safely. Eight caused flare-ups. They were bread, beef, eggs, sugar, pork, corn, milk and cheese."

Even though Llewellyn tested bread rather than separately testing its ingredients, he eventually discovered an elimination diet that worked successfully for him.

Confirming Allergies with Alternative Tests

Any of the tests described in this chapter may be used to confirm the results of other tests. For example, if the fasting test showed a sensitivity to beef, wheat and chocolate, you could confirm these results with the pulse and kinesiology tests.

Since neither the pulse nor kinesiology tests are as sensitive as the fasting test, I suggest using both methods to test your list of suspect foods. Then use the Food Elimination Test to check out any foods which tested allergy-positive.

If you have any doubts about foods you may eat in the future, you can give them a quick preliminary check out by the Quick Pulse Test or the Kinesiology method.

For greater certainty, you can also test any suspect food a second or third time, using the Quick Pulse Test or the Kinesiology method.

CHAPTER 9

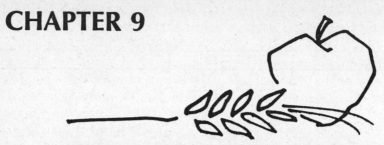

STRESSOR FOODS THAT PAVE THE WAY FOR ARTHRITIC DISEASE

The first step in recovering from any form of arthritic disease is to stop eating all Stressor Foods. Stressor Foods are those problem foods that tear down your health and pave the way for arthritis.

We call them Stressor Foods because they are so harmful to health that eating them places a stress on the body. When we continue to eat Stressor Foods over a period of years, the continued stress throws the body's self-regulatory systems out of balance and we become sickly and run down.

Healthy people don't get gout or arthritis because healthy people don't eat Stressor Foods.

Arthritic disease occurs only after years of harmful eating habits have led to physical di-stress in the joints and lowered the body's resistance.

How Good Is Your Health, Really?

The Holistic version of good health goes far beyond merely checking OK on a battery of diagnostic tests and being free of any discernible sign of disease.

"I always relied on my doctor to tell me how healthy I was," this was a 52-year old woman speaking. "He told me I was in good health. But a month later I was stricken by arthritis."

When I questioned Emily J. I learned that, despite her doctor's reassurance, she was far from being in optimum health when arthritis first appeared. Her diet consisted almost entirely of canned and convenience foods, white bread, fried dishes, and sugar-filled desserts.

As a result of the stress these foods had placed on her body, Emily J. was 25 pounds overweight, had frequent gastrointestinal distress, was unable to walk for more than ten minutes, and suffered from frequent colds and infections. Yet because she showed no symptoms of actual disease, her doctor had given Emily J. a clean bill of health.

Like virtually everyone who is stricken with arthritis, Emily J. was eating poorly. She had chronic constipation and frequent indigestion. By Holistic standards she was in mediocre health. But a medical check up had failed to find anything wrong.

Arthritis does not attack people in optimum health. It strikes only after years of eating Stressor Foods has caused a serious imbalance in body chemistry by raising cholesterol and fat levels, creating poor digestion and elimination, causing overweight and skeletal bone loss, and by causing di-stress in joints and making them a target for auto-immune attack triggered by food allergies.

Foods That Kill

Stressor Foods are the same killer foods that cause other degenerative diseases including heart disease, hypertension, diabetes and even some forms of cancer. No one can continue to eat Stressor Foods and remain permanently healthy.

The first step in recovery from gout or arthritis is to drop all Stressor Foods from the diet *now and for always!*

Stressor Foods Prevent Jerry B's Body from Healing Itself

Jerry B. didn't believe it was necessary to cut out Stressor Foods to recover from arthritis. Jerry had had rheumatoid arthritis for 5 years. He underwent food testing at an arthritis clinic and tested allergy-positive to wheat, beef, milk, potatoes, tomatoes and caffeine. Jerry stopped eating these allergenic foods and a few weeks later his arthritis began to disappear.

Although Jerry was told at the clinic to stop eating *all* Stressor Foods, he believed this wasn't really necessary.

"Why?" he asked himself. "I've stopped the foods I'm allergic to. My arthritis is gone."

But Jerry did not remain arthritis-free for long. Although some of the allergenic foods he had cut out were also Stressor Foods, he went right on eating other Stressor Foods. Nor did Jerry begin to eat the health-building Restorative Foods that would have made him well.

The result was that Jerry's nutritional stress remained uncorrected. Still out of balance, his immune system began to build an intolerance for other common foods that remained in his diet.

A few months after his arthritis cleared up, it was right back again.

As in Jerry's case, even though we stop eating all allergy-causing foods, if we remain nutritionally depleted by continuing to eat Stressor Foods, we may build new sensitivities to other common foods.

Our Chemicalized, Mass-Produced Imitation Food

The basic cause of arthritis are the Stressor Foods in our typical American diet. The foods that most of us are eating at every meal is slowly killing us.

Actually, it is not so much the food itself that makes us sick but the way it is raised and prepared. Our ancestors did not get heart disease because their meat came from wild game or from lean, unfattened steers bred on the range. Today, we eat marbled steaks from steers force-fed in fattening pens where they are routinely given hormones to make them fatter still.

Raw cow's milk seldom tests out allergy-positive. But modern homogenized milk contains an enzyme called Xanthine Oxidase that scars artery walls and heart tissue, causing cholesterol deposits and giving rise to hardening of the arteries, hypertension, strokes and heart attack. Homogenization also destroys the desirable enzyme Phosphatase plus essential B-vitamins and Vitamin C.

The wheat our ancestors ate was a perfectly wholesome food. But around 1900, millers discovered that refined flour would keep longer than whole wheat flour and bring in more profit. Refining destroys the germ of wheat, including all its fiber, and leaches out almost all vitamins and minerals. Prior to 1900, heart disease, appendicitis and hiatus hernia were rare. Today, diverticulosis—an ailment caused by refined foods and lack of fiber—is the most common disease in adult Americans while one of every two Americans over 50 suffer from varicose veins or hemorrhoids—other diseases caused by foods that lack fiber.

These same degenerative diseases, including gout and arthritis, appear in every country that adopts the western industrialized diet that most people eat in America. The plain fact is that 60 per cent of what most of us eat consists of just two foods: fat and sugar.

The western diet with its deadly amounts of fat and sugar, its distressing lack of fiber, and its proclivity for processed rather than whole foods has spread to every industrialized country. Until recently, the Japanese lived on a far more natural diet and their incidence of degenerative diseases, including gout and arthritis, was far below ours. But the Japanese are rapidly adopting the western diet and, as they do, their rate of arthritis, gout, heart disease, diabetes, and cancer has soared.

Counterfeit Foods—Our Disastrous Diet

Government statistics reveal the changing food picture in the U.S. In 1938, the average American ate 120 pounds of meat a year. Now we eat 160 pounds. Today, we eat 27 per cent fewer fresh vegetables and 39 per cent fewer fresh fruits than in 1938.

In the modern diet, more than half our food is processed, while such basic foods as meat and poultry are dangerously tampered with long before they reach the processing stage.

Research shows that almost everyone who suffers from arthritis or gout is a heavy eater of refined carbohydrates (white flour and sugar) and foods dangerously high in saturated fats such as dairy products, seafood, steak, eggs and other forms of animal protein. Many arthritis patients are also steady consumers of fast, convenience foods.

The same research also shows that most black Africans, who eat no refined foods at all and who live entirely on fresh, whole natural foods, seldom suffer from gout or arthritis or from any other degenerative disease.

The same is true among vegetarians in the U.S. True vegetarians, those who not only abstain from rich meats but also from eggs and fat-laden dairy foods, scarcely if ever experience any form of arthritic disease. Nor do they often get heart disease, diabetes, cancer, osteoporosis, diverticulosis, varicose veins, appendicitis, hiatus hernia and the long melancholy litany of other degenerative diseases all caused by Stressor Foods.

As the Africans and vegetarians prove, when we feed our bodies the kind of natural foods on which man thrived over millions of years, we remain healthy and free of disease. But overloading our digestive tract with rich fats, animal proteins and refined foods is like feeding gasoline to a wood stove.

Our bodies are simply not adapted to the foods we eat today. When we insist on punishing our bodies with Stressor Foods, it's like buying a one-way ticket to self-destruction.

The U.S. Government Recognizes the Risks of Stressor Foods

The U.S. Government itself recommends a drastic reduction in the Stressor Foods in our diet. When the Senate's Select Committee on Nutrition and Human Needs issued its *Dietary Goals for the U.S.* a few years ago, its six principal recommendations involved a significant reduction in fats and refined foods.

The *Alternative Diet Book* published by the National Institutes of Health recommends major reductions in meat, egg yolks, lard, organ meats, buttermilk, poultry skin, dairy products and all forms of saturated (animal) fats. This U.S. Government dietary guide recommends that meat and poultry should be used only as condiments to a natural diet of grains and vegetables. It recommends cutting down the excessive amounts of animal protein with which most of us overload our liver-pancreas systems and reducing protein intake to only 3–4 ounces daily. Fish and poultry, it says, are safer foods than meat.

Again, in 1977, the prestigious Worldwatch Institute of Washington, D.C. released a report it had prepared for the United Nations that linked the conventional American diet with six of the ten leading causes of death in the U.S.

Literally hundreds of similar studies carried out in every country from Finland to England, Israel and Japan say the same thing.

For all degenerative diseases begin in the same way: through nutritional stress that distorts the carbohydrate metabolism in the liver-pancreas system. When this key self-regulatory system throws the circulatory system off balance, we get heart disease and hypertension. When it distorts our fat-insulin balance, we get diabetes. When it suppresses the immune system, we get cancer. When it creates a dysfunction in the digestive system, we get diverticulosis. When an abnormality appears in calcium metabolism, we get bone loss or osteoporosis.

Among all degenerative diseases is arthritis the *only* exception? The facts show that it is not.

When the immune system is distorted, we get rheumatoid and similar forms of arthritis together with a variety of related auto-immune diseases. When we eat fat-laden Stressor Foods and become overweight, we get osteo-arthritis. When we become overweight and eat rich foods high in purines, we get gout.

The evidence is clear and unmistakable. The message of almost all modern nutritional research is to cut down on all fats, refined foods and excessive animal protein—the Stressor Foods.

Alice W. Recovers from Double Arthritis When She Eliminates All Stressor Foods

How successful this step can be was demonstrated when I met Alice W. at a Florida mobile home park. Lean, suntanned and athletic, at 58 Alice looked a glowing picture of robust health. But ten years earlier, she had been diagnosed as having both osteo and rheumatoid arthritis.

"I was so weak, I could scarcely open a door," she told me. "Each morning, my hands and fingers were so stiff I had to soak them in hot water before I could dress. I was in constant pain and my doctor had prescribed the maximum dosage of steroids.

"I was forty pounds overweight, but the doctor never mentioned diet. I went right on drinking six colas each day and stuffing myself full of hamburgers, hot dogs, white bread, ice cream and cheese.

"The doctor told me I would never recover, so I began reading nutritional magazines. I soon discovered there *were* alternatives to drugs. I also learned I'd have to act fast if I were ever to get better. So I took the plunge and enrolled at a Natural Hygiene institution."

Alice paused to explain that Natural Hygiene—meaning the Science of Natural Health—is the original Holistic health care system.

"The Hygienists use fasting for purification but do not test foods for allergies," she said. "They started me out with a five day water fast, then put me on a diet that cut out just about all fats, refined foods and animal protein. The only fats I ate were in seeds, nuts and avocadoes. And I got all my protein from vegetable sources.

"Well, by the fifth day of the fast at least half of my pain had gone. The Hygienist doctor told me I must gradually lose weight and that a diet of fresh, living natural foods would restore my health to normal.

"Week by week, I gradually lost weight without dieting or feeling hungry. In eight weeks time, just as my weight reached normal, the last of the arthritis symptoms vanished.

"Since then, I've strictly avoided all fats, refined foods and animal protein. The arthritis never came back. And that Hygienic diet of living foods is so zestful and revitalizing that, every year since, I've reached a new high plateau of health and wellness."

Learning to Recognize Stressor Foods

How do we recognize a Stressor Food? To do so, we must learn a few simple facts concerning nutrition. All foods fall into three types: fats, proteins and carbohydrates.

FATS

Fats are divided into two classes:

Saturated Fats: are so-called because each of their carbon atoms are saturated with all the hydrogen they can hold. Saturated fats are hard or solid at room temperature, are of animal origin and contain cholesterol. Some foods rich in saturated fats are high-grade meats, organ meats, egg yolks, seafood, shellfish, whole milk dairy products, lard and poultry skin.

Poly-unsaturated Fats: have room to absorb more hydrogen. They are liquid at room temperature, of vegetable origin and contain no cholesterol. Typical poly-unsaturated fats are vegetable oils like safflower, soybean, sunflower, cottonseed, sesame and corn oils. (Peanut oil and olive oil are mono-saturated fats and are also cholesterol-free.)

Atherosclerosis, or hardening of the arteries, is caused when cholesterol in saturated fats is deposited in the arteries like rust in a waterpipe, gradually blocking off oxygen and other essential nutrients to joints, heart, brain and other organs. The result is di-stress in the joints together with severe risk of heart attack, stroke or hypertension.

Research has also shown that not all cholesterol is dangerous. Only cholesterol with a Low Density Lipoprotein fraction (LDL) causes artherosclerosis. Cholesterol with a High Density Lipoprotein fraction (HDL) actually helps sweep cholesterol deposits out of the arteries.

Poly- or mono-unsaturated fats are also cholesterol-free and, therefore, do not harm arteries. These unsaturated fats also help create a High Density Lipoprotein fraction that prevents LDL-cholesterol from clogging arteries.

By comparison to saturated fats which distort body chemistry and cause atherosclerosis, arthritis and various killer diseases, unsaturated fats are relatively harmless.

Processing Makes Safe Foods Dangerous

But—and wouldn't you know it—the food processing industry has found a way to make these vegetable oils highly dangerous. They have discovered how to inject these oils with more hydrogen to turn them into Trans-Acids that are hard and solid at room temperature just like saturated fats.

Be warned: hydrogenated, or partially-hydrogenated vegetable oils are more dangerous than saturated fats. They are not natural foods and are considered the most potentially dangerous of all foods. These fats are widely used in margarine, factory breads, salad oils, mayonnaise, snack foods and just about all processed foods.

A recent University of Maryland study that correlated fats in the human diet with increased risk of cancer made special mention of the extra hazards of partially-hydrogenated vegetable oils. Oils are hydrogenated to give them longer shelf life and to make them more profitable to the manufacturer. In doing so, of course, they shorten millions of human lives.

This isn't to say you should go overboard on plain vegetable oils either. They are also a processed food. Many nutritionists believe that they soon turn rancid without any noticeable change in taste and that this rancidity can cause cancer. But cold-pressed, freshly-squeezed oils are free of this risk for a day or two if kept refrigerated.

However, the ideal way to eat fat is to simply eat the seeds from which vegetables oils are made. In any case, the body can synthesize all the fat it needs from other foods. Our actual daily need for fat is so low it could be met by a bowl of oatmeal or an ear of corn.

Fats of all types can contribute to diseases like diabetes, and fats are one of the two principal culprits that throw our carbohydrate metabolism out of balance and set the stage for arthritic disease. So the fewer saturated fats and processed oils we eat, the better. The safest sources of fat are fresh, whole seeds, nuts and avocadoes.

Stored-Up Food Poisons Cause Arthritic Disease

Saturated fats carry an extra danger signal. All animal fats have a proclivity for storing toxic petro-chemicals, drugs used in animal feeds, and other poisons. The greater the fat content of any animal food, the greater the residue of chemical pesticides, insecticides, herbicides and fertilizers stored in it. The higher up the food chain, the greater the risk. Many fruits and vegetables are sprayed as many as a dozen times before harvesting. When eaten by animals, poultry or fish, the pesticides on these plants become concentrated in their tissue at 13 times the original level in the plant.

When an osprey, pelican or eagle eats a fish in one of our rivers or estuaries, the concentration of chlorinated hydrocarbons in its tissues reaches such toxic levels that the birds can no longer reproduce. You can imagine how these deadly poisons can unbalance our entire body chemistry.

This is why we recommend eating only deep ocean fish and not fish or seafood from our rivers, lakes, coasts and estuaries. Almost all are contaminated by agricultural run-off and industrial pollutants.

You probably never thought of cod or haddock as wild

game. But these low-fat, deep-ocean fish are the last uncontaminated wild game readily available. If you've ever wondered why Eskimo in their native habitat do not get degenerative diseases despite all the meat and fish they eat, the reason is that they eat only wild game. Compared to the lethally high-fat content of commercially-raised cattle, wild game such as whales, seals and caribou have a comparatively low fat concentration. For most us, cod and haddock is the closest we can get to eating wild game.

Besides creating blood vessel damage and inhibiting the function of insulin, fat also causes increased sensitivity to certain foods. It also causes di-stress in joints by separating tendons and ligaments, thereby creating tension on ligaments surrounding a joint.

A high-fat diet is the surest route to gout and arthritis.

Stressor Foods Are Pernicious to Health

You may have read recent articles denying that cholesterol is a cause of heart disease and saying that it's all right to go on eating foods rich in saturated fats. The articles say that it is not merely cholesterol but cholesterol with a Low Density Lipoprotein fraction that is responsible for hardening of the arteries and heart disease, and that much of our cholesterol is synthesized by the liver. If we don't get the cholesterol we need from food, the liver will produce it for us.

What the articles don't say is that cholesterol synthesized by the body tends to have a High Density Lipoprotein fraction—the type of cholesterol that does not cause heart disease. Thus the less cholesterol you eat in food—much of which is the bad LDL type—the more our liver manufactures of the good HDL type.

Most organizations doing research on heart disease have repudiated claims endorsing a high-fat diet. Regardless of pet theories you may read, the less fat in your diet the safer you are from gout and arthritis and all other types of degenerative disease.

Most Holistically-oriented nutritionists recommend that you derive an absolute maximum of 20 per cent of your calories from fat and that you would be better off with one half or one fourth this amount.

PROTEIN

Protein is the building block of cells and tissue. It consists of 22 amino acids of which the body can synthesize only 14. The remaining 8 (some nutritionists say ten) are called Essential Amino Acids and must be obtained directly from foods. Virtually all animal-derived foods (including fish, poultry, dairy products and eggs) contain whole protein which includes the 8 Essential Amino Acids.

Protein can also be supplied by vegetables, grains, nuts and seeds. But no single vegetarian foods supplies whole protein. Vegetarians complement one protein-containing food with two or three others to obtain all 8 Essential Amino Acids at a single meal. Since protein cannot be stored in the body, all 8 Essential Amino Acids must be eaten together to produce whole protein.

The problem with animal protein is that you can easily eat too much, thereby creating four arthritis-causing effects. First, an excessive protein intake creates an imbalance in carbohydrate metabolism. Second, it increases the amount of protein food particles in the bloodstream. Protein fragments are much more likely to be recognized as foreign antigens than other types of foods.

Third, with very few exceptions, to eat animal protein such as steak or liver, you must eat the high-fat content that comes along with it. And fourth, studies have shown that a high-protein diet causes bone loss at twice the normal rate. Since all persons with arthritis are deficient in calcium, the stuff of which bones are made, anything which accelerates bone loss is extremely undesirable.

The body's actual requirements for protein are amazingly small. A 160-pound man needs only 2½ ounces of whole protein daily. Hence many Holistically-oriented nutritionists recommend that we derive a maximum of 15 per cent of our calories from protein. Many believe we would be better off with only ten per cent.

CARBOHYDRATES

Carboydrates include almost all fruits, vegetables and grains and are our main source of energy. Carbohydrates have been given a bad name by writers of fad diet books to the extent that nearly everyone today believes that carbohydrates are fattening.

Not so! There are good and bad carbohydrates. And good carbohydrates—even those containing starch—are far from fattening.

The Good Carbohydrates

Good carbohydrates, called *Complex, Unrefined Carbohydrates*, consist of whole, fresh fruits, vegetables and grains as they come off the tree or out of the ground. Complex carbohydrates are all living foods (as also are nuts and seeds) that, if planted in the ground will grow into a plant or tree.

They are called "complex" because the living cells of these foods are encased in walls of cellulose. Cellulose cannot be digested by humans. It passes through the digestive system as fiber. All complex carbohydrates are high in fiber.

Because cellulose cannot be digested, the cell walls of complex carbohydrates decompose slowly, allowing the carbohydrates inside to enter the bloodstream at a slow, gradual pace without upsetting the equilibrium of the body's self-regulatory systems.

The Bad Carbohydrates

Bad carbohydrates are called *Simple, Refined Carbohydrates*. They were originally complex carbohydrates, such as sugar or grains, that have been highly refined during milling. In refining, both the kernel and all fiber, vitamins, minerals and enzymes are destroyed along with the cell walls, leaving nothing but hollow calories and zero nutrition.

Without cellulose walls, refined carbohydrates are rapidly absorbed into the bloodstream. The sudden flush of sugar into which they are converted sends blood fat and blood sugar levels soaring. Many heart specialists believe refined carbohydrates are as threatening to patients with heart disease as saturated fats or hydrogenated vegetable oils.

The most common refined carbohydrates are sugar, white flour and hulled, white rice. Because cereals like wheat are highly refined into tiny particles, they are readily absorbed from the digestive tract into the bloodstream. This fact alone makes refined wheat flour the most common of all food allergens.

Most Holistically oriented nutritionists believe that 80 per cent of our calories should come from complex carbohydrates and none at all from simple, refined carbohydrates. Several nutritionists have suggested that simple, refined carbohydrates are so menacing to health they should carry a warning sign like cigarettes.

CHAPTER 10

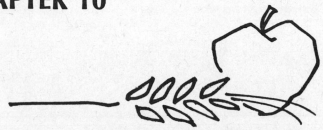

THE STRESSOR FOODS THAT BLOCK THE HEALING OF GOUT AND ARTHRITIS

All Stressor Foods but eggs are dead foods. If you planted them in the ground, they would *not* grow into living plants. These lifeless foods which, of course, include meat, fish and poultry have another common drawback. They are totally devoid of enzymes.

Enzymes are health-promoting food components that in fresh, living foods aid digestion by acting as catalysts. When dead foods are eaten, all digestive enzymes must be produced by the pancreas and other organs. This stressful task helps unbalance the body's self-regulatory liver-pancreas system and lays the groundwork for arthritic disease.

All canned, packaged, preserved, processed, manufactured and convenience foods are dead and lifeless with all their health-restoring enzymes destroyed and most of their vitamin and mineral content depleted. Many frozen foods are also partially pre-cooked and are nutritionally empty and hollow.

Many foods are processed simply to give them longer shelf life. Yet no thought is ever given to extending the life of the consumer. All processed foods are Stressor Foods and should be ruthlessly discarded from the diet.

Pseudo Foods—A Travesty of Real Foods

Good health-promoting foods seldom come in boxes, packages, jars or cans. Nor are they cut up or fragmented in any way. The only wholesome potatoes are whole potatoes in exactly the same state as they were dug from the ground with their skins intact and with sprouts budding out to prove they are still alive and have not been sprayed. Potatoes that are cut up or are not whole are pseudo foods: instant mashed potatoes, French fries, potato chips, hashed browns, you name them—all are nutritional disasters guaranteed to hasten arthritis and other diseases.

Any food which is not whole, fresh, raw and completely natural is a Stressor Food. Any food that has been processed in any way or that has been tampered with while growing is a Stressor Food.

There may be a few exceptions like bread made exclusively of 100 per cent whole grain flour and entirely free of fats, sugar and chemical additives. These we'll try to point out as we go along.

How to Stop Committing Supermarket Suicide

Don't be misled into thinking that refined foods are OK after they've been fortified or enriched. Manufacturers may replace a few of the vitamins and minerals they've destroyed in refining. But the foods are still devoid of all enzymes and fiber.

Supermarket shelves abound with boxes and packages of counterfeit foods which bear long lists of the many vitamins and minerals they supposedly contain. The lists may sound impressive, but the foods still contain chemical preservatives and artificial coloring or flavor. And their fiber and protein content is often completely devitalized.

Don't be fooled by containers which state "no artificial anything." Actually, the manufacturer is telling the truth. All the anti-oxidants, emulsifiers, anti-bacterial agents, bleachers, blenders, anti-caking and anti-fungal agents that each food contains are not artificial. They are real, honest-to-goodness chemical additives.

Take a cold, hard look at any food container labelled "All

Natural Ingredients" or "No artificial preservatives added."
Wholesome, health-building foods rarely come in boxes, cans,
jars or packages. The preservatives these foods contain are not
artificial. They are real bonafide chemical preservatives.

Jars of jam or preserves labelled "no artificial preservatives"
state the literal truth. What they don't tell you is that the high
sugar content of the fruit itself preserves the jam. In doing so, it
destroys all nutritional value along with the fiber.

Other than freezing in which absolutely no chemicals are
used, drying is the only natural way to preserve foods. Even that
is second choice.

In drying, foods like dates, figs and raisins lose their cell
walls. When eaten, they produce the same flush of sugar in the
bloodstream as do refined carbohydrates. A few dried fruits can
be safely eaten from time to time. Small amounts of raisins
mixed with nuts or seeds, or used for similar flavoring, can be
eaten daily. But frequent binges of dried fruits in large amounts
is another nutritional No No.

To sum up: The food processing industry created the modern Western Diet. As this devitalized diet was adopted, the
incidence of heart disease, colon and breast cancer, diabetes,
osteoporosis, and gout and arthritis all increased right in step.

Just because everyone else goes on eating this harmful
Western Diet, you don't have to.

To avoid it, totally ignore the row upon row of cans, boxes,
jars and packaged foods that line your supermarket shelves.
Shop instead in the produce section. By cutting out dead foods
from your diet and replacing them with fresh, living foods, you
can transform your present harmful, modern diet into the same
health-building, primitive diet on which the human body has
thrived for millennnia.

Rebecca S. Discovers That
Arthritis Is the Junk Food Disease

It was difficult to believe that the tireless, radiantly healthy
woman who had just given me a thorough trouncing on the
tennis court was crippled with arthritis until 8 years ago.

"The pain first appeared in my back and ribs when I was
fifty-four," Rebecca S. told me after the game. "I visited a
number of doctors. None could do anything. In the end I spent a

week at a diagnostic clinic. They said I had osteo-arthritis of the spine and that it was incurable.

"From then on life became an endless round of aspirin and constant, miserable pain. I still can't believe that I put up with that constant agony for three whole years.

"No one at the clinic told me that being overweight was half the cause. Or that all the fat and sugar I was eating had any effect on arthritis. At last, a friend suggested I see an herbalist.

"Well, the herbalist, a very knowledgeable German lady, said I was too far gone for herbs to help much. She said if I were ever to get well I'd better decide to help myself right now. She told me about what she called orthomolecular therapy. That means treating disease with food.

"She said I must stop eating dead foods like fats, sugar and refined flour as well as foods of animal origin, and stimulants. I was to eat nothing but fresh, natural living foods instead.

"The pain and aspirin had me so frustrated I was ready to clutch at anything. I followed her advice exactly.

"Slowly, a bit at a time, I did begin to feel better. After six weeks, I'd lost twelve pounds and the pain in my back was definitely fading. I could walk and do housework again.

"I had to lose eighteen more pounds before the pain ended. My back was still filled with calcium deposits. Every time I moved, they cracked and groaned. The German lady taught me yoga bending exercises. Every day I'd bend my spine easily and gently in every direction. I could hear the calcium cracking and breaking up. Eventually, it was all absorbed.

"But I'd still have an occasional flare-up. The lady tested my pulse and found I was allergic to corn, potatoes and tomatoes. As soon as I dropped these foods, the flare-ups stopped coming back.

"Now I can walk five miles, swim for an hour or play tennis half the day. I do eat some corn, potatoes and tomatoes on a rotational basis once a week. But I never eat anything that contains fat, refined foods, animal protein, alcohol or caffeine. All my friends still eat these lifeless foods. But I'm the only one who is completely healthy and free of any chronic disease."

Stressor Foods You Should Never Eat Again

Here, as a guide to what foods to avoid, is a brief run down on some of the most stressful foods.

ALCOHOL: Hundreds of doctors and orthodox nutritionists still believe the myth that a moderate amount of alcohol will lower blood pressure and is beneficial for older people. Any blood pressure drop is merely temporary. Alcohol depletes the body's supply of B-vitamins and paves the way for arthritis by interfering with the body's self-regulatory systems.

BREAD: Bleached white flour is minus its germ and bran and is just another zero-nutrition food. But most factory-made "whole wheat" bread is also fake. If you examine the label closely, it usually reads "Made WITH 100 per cent whole grain flour." Instead of being made exclusively OF whole grain (unrefined) flour, the bread also probably contains large amounts of refined flour as well as sugar, eggs, hydrogenated vegetable oil, dairy products and chemical additives.

CAFFEINE is a legal shot of speed that creates a "high" by distorting the output of the adrenal glands—an essential link in the body's self-regulatory systems. Whether in coffee, cocoa, chocolate, cola drinks or tea, caffeine is a highly addictive food that invariably tests allergy-positive.

You can easily overcome its addiction by each day replacing one cup of coffee with a cup of tea. Tea has half the caffeine content of coffee. If your daily quota is 7 cups of coffee, in one week you can replace it with 7 cups of tea and cut your caffeine intake by half. The following week, replace one cup of tea per day with a cup of herb tea or carob. In 14 days, you will have overcome the caffeine habit completely.

Caffeine is also a vitamin antagonist and is often taken with sugar and cream—two other Stressor Foods.

CHEMICAL ADDITIVES: Anyone who eats the conventional American way takes 4–5 pounds of toxic chemical additives into the body each year. Despite the banning of a few dyes and other dangerous additives by the FDA, 3,000 additives remain in use.

The majority have not been tested for safety by the FDA. Their safety is determined by the food processing industry itself, often in laboratories subsidized by the manufacturers. Stored in body fat, these poisons hasten arthritis by causing imbalances in our self-regulatory systems. Many are also known to cause cancer.

Some brands of ice cream and diet sodas may consist 50 per cent of chemical additives. Almost every processed food contains a host of nitrites, coloring, stabilizers, bleaching agents, texturing agents, emulsifiers and other chemicals, few of which have ever been tested for their long term danger to human life. Texturing agents make limp canned vegetables appear crisp and fresh. Flavoring agents mask a disagreeable taste. Even a wholesome food like yogurt often contains Stressor Foods like gelatin, sugar and artificial fruit flavors.

CONDIMENTS exist only to mask the disagreeable taste of other Stressor Foods. If a conventional food needs its taste disguised, isn't it time to ask what is so great about hamburger, hot dogs, liver, French fries or sausages that are customarily smothered in ketchup or Worcestershire sauce?

Undoubtedly, the worst condiment is MSG (mono-sodium glutamate) widely used in cooking at cafeterias and Chinese restaurants to supposedly enhance taste. After eating MSG-doped food, thousands of people have discovered the MSG syndrome—headaches, stiffness in the neck, jaw and other joints, and numbness in the limbs.

All commercial sauces and pickles, ketchup, mustard, pepper, vinegar, salad dressings, mayonnaise and other condiments are Stressor Foods. Piquant sauces inflame the stomach lining and increase the rate at which particles of allergenic foods enter the bloodstream. All condiments are harmful and many indirectly pave the way for gout or arthritis.

Salt, for example, can cause arthritis symptoms by creating edema in joints.

Throw out all these foodless foods and replace them with natural herb seasonings, garlic, onion or lemon.

COW'S MILK is fine for calves. But millions of children and adults are unable to tolerate the lactose, fat or protein in milk. Many older people cannot break down the calcium in milk and this leads to osteoporosis and arthritis. The same intolerance may extend to dairy products like cream or cheese. Seventy per cent of blacks have difficulty digesting milk. Cow's milk and its products are also a major arthritis-causing allergen.

However, if you have no sensitivity to them, low-fat cottage cheese or low-fat yogurt, when entirely free of other Stressor Foods or additives, are sound health-restoring foods.

SUGAR is omni-present in almost all processed foods. Most Americans consume two pounds of this stressful food each week. Sugar causes the blood sugar level to soar. Then just as suddenly, it plummets and gives you a letdown. In doing so, it upsets both the liver-pancreas system and the action of the adrenal glands in the hormone-endocrine system. When thrown off balance by eating sugar, these key self-regulatory systems transfer their stress to the immune system, opening the way for arthritic disease.

Most brown sugar is simply white sugar coated with molasses, while turbanide sugar is partially refined. Not recommended is saccharine or any other synthetic sweetener. Nor is extracted fructose recommended as a sugar substitute.

The best sweetener is no sweetener at all. However, if you must have a substitute, blackstrap molasses is the best alternative. It is rich in B-vitamins, iron and other minerals. Honey that is raw, unfiltered and unheated can also be used in small amounts in place of sugar.

Even though nutritionally more desirable than sugar, these sweeteners can have the same effect on body chemistry as sugar. If you must have something sweet, try a few dates, figs or raisins, some sweet, fresh fruits or freshly-squeezed fruit juice or sweet vegetables like baked yams or carrots.

Pain Folds Its Fangs When Ella C. Stops Eating Stressor Foods

Can you imagine anyone being grateful for having a heart attack?

Ella C. is. At 58, Ella began suffering with osteo-arthritis pain in the hips and knees.

But hear her story in her own words.

"I was overweight and the pain in my hips was so severe that only a shot of Novocaine could bring relief. My rheumatologist said it was progressive and at my age would never improve.

"My diet was full of fat, and I snacked on sugar-filled foods all day. Yet I was never advised to change my diet.

"The following year I had a heart attack. Fortunately it was just a mild one. As a result, I came under the care of a cardiologist. He was appalled at my diet.

"He cut out all of the fat, sugar, meats and dairy foods I loved. He said if I didn't stick to the diet I'd have another heart attack soon and this one would be fatal.

"As you can imagine, I stuck right with that diet. Instead of the fat and sugar, I ate fresh fruit and vegetable salads. I soon came to love the honest taste of these living foods and I used no condiments at all.

"It took three months for my weight to drop back to normal. Every week, as my weight went down, my arthritis also began to disappear. On the day my weight reached normal, the last of my arthritis symptoms vanished.

"The cardiologist said mine was one of several cases he'd seen where a person had changed their diet to recover from heart disease and then found that the same diet brought recovery from arthritis or gout.

"He said that the cholesterol that was clogging the arteries to my heart also blocked the flow of blood and nutrients to my knees and hips.

"When I got rid of the cause of arthritis, the fat and sugar and other junk that made me overweight and clogged my arteries, my body healed itself. But if I'd never had the heart attack, I'd still be suffering with arthritis today."

Ella C. is now a hale and hearty 68 and has been totally free of both arthritis and heart disease symptoms for more than 8 years.

Profile of Peril—
The Worst Foods You Can Eat

This is a nearly complete list of all Stressor Foods that cause nutritional distress and that lead, eventually, to arthritis, gout and other degenerative diseases. Whether or not you have arthritis or gout, to attain optimum health all should be totally excluded from the diet on a lifelong basis. The list is in addition to other Stressor Foods already mentioned in this chapter.

The list refers only to commercial products. Health food stores often carry more acceptable forms of some foods. Too, some of these foods can be prepared at home with more wholesome ingredients.

Alcohol	Baked beans
Anchovies	Bakery products
Artificial dairy foods	Beef (prime)
Artifical sweeteners	Beef tallow
Baby foods	Beer
Bacon	Blue cheese

Bouillon
Brains
Bread (commercial)
Breakfast cereals
   (containing sugar)
Broth
Brown sugar
Butter
Butterfat
Cakes
Cake mixes
Calcium propionate
Candy
Canned foods
Carbonated drinks
Cheese (except skim milk
   cheeses)
Chili sauce
Chocolate
Chow mein
Clams
Cocoa
Cocktail snacks
Coffee
Cola drinks
Convenience foods
Crab
Crackers
Cream
Cruellers
Dairy foods (whole milk)
Dairy substitutes
Diet sodas and colas
Doughnuts
Dry drink powders
Duck
Egg noodles
Egg yokes
Fast foods
Fat (all forms except in
   seeds, nuts and
   avocados)

Fatty fish
Fatty meats
Fish roe
Flour (refined, bleached,
   enriched)
Frankfurters
French fries
Fried foods
Fried rice mixtures
Frozen desserts
Frozen dinners
Frozen pre-cooked foods
Frozen yogurt
Fruit yogurt
Gelatin
Goose
Gravies
Ham
Hamburger
Heart
Herring
High-grade meats
Honey (processed)
Hot dogs
Hot sauces
Hot spices
Hydrogenated or partially
   hydrogenated vegetable
   oils
Ice cream
Ice milk
Instant breakfasts
Instant foods (all types)
Jams
Jellies
Jello
Ketchup
Kidneys
Lard
Lights (lungs)
Liquor
Liver

Lobster
Luncheon meats
Marbled meats
Margarine
Marmalade
Mayonnaise
Meat (red, fatty)
Meat soup
Milk (homogenized whole
  cow's milk)
Monosodium glutamate
  (MSG)
Mustard
Nitrates, nitrites
Non-dairy creamers
Noodles
Organ meats
Oysters
Paté de foie gras
Pasta (refined)
Pastry
Pork
Potatoes (flakes, chips,
  processed)
Poultry skin
Powdered whole milk
Prepared mixes
Pre-prepared main dishes,
  desserts, etc.
Preserves
Puddings
Pudding mixes
Quick-preparation foods
  (all types)
Red meats

Rice (refined, hulled)
Salad dressings
Salt
Sardines
Sausage
Scallops
Scrabble
Seafood
Shellfish
Sherbert
Shortening
Shrimp
Smoked foods
Snack foods
Soft drinks
Soup
Sour cream
Spaghetti (refined)
Spare ribs
Steak
Suet
Sugar
Sweetbreads
Tea (caffeine-containing)
Tobacco smoke
Tongue
Tunafish (canned)
Turbanide sugar
TV dinners
Vinegar
White bread
White flour
White rice
Wine

Cutting Out Stressor Foods
Ends John L's Nagging Gout

"I was racked with constant, throbbing pain," is how 53-year old John L. described his gout. "My toes and insteps were excruciatingly tender, and the flesh over the joints had turned hard, shiny and purple.

"My doctor told me it was caused by purines in certain foods. He said it was easier to control gout with drugs than to bother going on a diet. But the drugs gave me itchy skin, headaches, abdominal pain and diarrhea. For me, the cure was as bad as the disease.

"Finally, I went to a nutritionist. He put me on a five-day water fast. Then I had to cut out all foods that contained purines.

"In just two weeks, the pain and inflammation in my joints subsided. But I still continued to have minor flare-ups. The nutritionist said these are due to my being overweight. He said that if I dropped my weight back to normal they would disappear."

John L. did eventually lose weight, and the rest of his gout disappeared along with the surplus pounds.

As John L. discovered, most doctors today treat gout with drugs instead of diet. The reason given is that patients will usually not stick to their diet. Also most gout sufferers are overweight. To become completely gout-free, weight must be reduced to normal.

Forbidden Foods for Those with Gout

Gout is actually caused by an excess of purines in the diet. Purines are the basic substance of uric acid. They abound in such rich foods as shellfish, organ meats, goose, caviar and other oily, fatty delicacies.

Until purine-rich foods are totally eliminated from the diet, gout cannot be reversed. Here is a list of the purine-rich foods that John L. was forbidden to eat:

Alcohol	Goose
Anchovies	Gravies
Beef tongue	Herring
Bouillon	Kidneys
Brains	Liver
Caviar	Mackeral
Clams	Meat soup
Coffee	Organ meats
Duck	Oysters
Fish roe	Pork

Sardines	Soft drinks
Sausage	Squab
Scrabble	Sugar
Shellfish	Sweetbreads
Shrimp	Yeast

It is absolutely vital, in any case of gout, to eliminate every last one of these foods totally, immediately and for always. Right after that, cut out all of the Stressor Foods.

How to Immunize Yourself Against Gout, Arthritis and All Killer Diseases

Regardless what type of arthritic disease you have—or even if you do not have arthritic disease—you should strictly avoid all Stressor Foods *for the rest of your life.* These life-threatening foods pave the way for *all* types of degenerative disease, not merely gout or arthritis.

Eliminate these foods entirely and you will have virtually immunized yourself against not only gout or arthritis but also heart disease, hypertension, diabetes, osteoporosis, diverticulosis, kidney disease and other killer diseases that flourish wherever the Western Diet has appeared.

CHAPTER 11

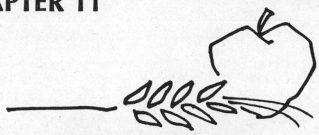

THE INCREDIBLE ARTHRITIS-HEALING POWERS OF RESTORATIVE FOODS

The body is self-healing when the *cause* of disease is removed. This is the Holistic Law of Healing.

We have removed the cause of arthritic disease—the Stressor Foods that stress the joints with overweight and poor nutrition and the Allergy Foods which trigger the immune system to harass the cells in our di-stressed joints.

But let's always remember that arthritis itself is nothing more than the body's way of responding to this stress and attack. The pain, stiffness and inflammation of gout and arthritis are all responses by the body as it attempts to defend itself.

The body itself creates gout and arthritis. Therefore, the body itself can heal gout and arthritis.

To do so, we have only to remove the cause—the Stressor and Allergy Foods—and to replace them with Restorative Foods that can rebuild the body's ailing nutrition and restore its chemical balance.

Undoubtedly, after reading the list of Stressor Foods that are now forbidden, you are probably wondering what there is left to eat. How about:

- **The entire vegetable kingdom:** that is, every single fruit, vegetable, bean and spout in existence; also soybean products like tofu and tempeh.

153

- **The entire grain kingdom:** that is, the whole spectrum of cereals and grains provided they are unrefined.

- **All nuts and seed.** Excluding only the coconut, all nuts and seeds are rich in nutrients the body needs to heal itself.

- **Low-fat foods of animal origin** such as ocean fish, egg whites, lean meats and low-fat dairy foods.

At any supermarket produce counter, you have a choice of at least 12 and up to 20 different vegetables and a dozen different fruits depending on season. Most supermarkets carry at least half a dozen varieties of dried beans as well as a choice of whole grains, dried fruits and unsalted nuts.

Elsewhere in your supermarket you'll find frozen deep sea fish, lean meats like veal, and low-fat cheese and yogurt.

Most granaries and health food stores offer at least a dozen different unsprayed grains. Many carry up to 20 or more varieties together with a dozen different types of beans, eight or more varieties of nuts, several different seeds for eating, and a variety of seeds and grains for sprouting. These stores also often carry breads made entirely from whole grains and free of fats, sugar, hydrogenated oils and other destructive foods.

They stock low-fat dairy foods and some even have barnyard chickens, raw milk and wild game.

Finding Super Nutrition in Your Supermarket

In their whole, natural form exactly as they come from the tree, the ground, the animal or from the ocean, these Restorative Foods will supply your body with all the nutrients it needs to rebuild di-stressed joints and restore high-level wellness.

(A very few exceptions like low-fat dairy foods and tofu have been mildly processed; beans, raisins and dates have been dried; and meat and fish have been frozen. But all other Restorative Foods are fresh and alive.)

Even dried beans are alive, and yogurt contains living bacteria. Every fresh, raw fruit, vegetable, grain, nut and seed is still living. All grains, nuts, seeds and fruits, as well as vegetables like potatoes, will sprout and grow if planted in the ground. The cells in green, leafy vegetables continue to live until the leaves wilt and droop.

Rabbit food, I hear someone say. Well, wouldn't you rather be a healthy, active rabbit than a carnivore crippled with gout or arthritis? Dead foods make listless, lifeless people prone to disease. At least 90 per cent of Restorative Foods are fresh and alive shortly before eating. The reason is that they are grown, not manufactured. All their health-building chlorophyll, vitamins, minerals, enzymes and fiber are still intact.

The Holistic Healing Values of Certain Common Fruits and Vegetables

Many of Nature's Restorative Foods are so commonplace that their nutritional healing values have been overlooked. But all vegetables, fruits, grains, nuts and seeds are natural foods that work Holistically to bring about positive changes in both mind and body. And to ensure total health, nutrition must be viewed in terms of the Whole Person rather than in terms of trying to cure a specific disease.

So let's not underestimate the value of whole, simple, natural foods. Some very plain jane fruits and vegetables are making news in scientific circles for their healing and protective qualities. And if natural foods hadn't made people feel better, they would never have achieved their present popularity.

Guidelines for Eating Away Gout and Arthritis

- Buy and eat only whole, fresh, raw, still-living foods in their natural, unprocessed state free of salt and additives. This means that you buy only fresh, raw fruits and vegetables, whole grains, and whole nuts and seeds—unchanged in any way by man and exactly as Nature produced them.

- Eat as many foods as possible uncooked and uncut. If you cannot chew raw vegetables, nuts or seeds, then cut them up or grind them just before eating. But if your teeth are good, serve as many foods as possible whole and unfragmented. This way, they retain all their enzymes, vitamins and fiber without loss.

- Avoid cooking any foods you can enjoy eating raw. Foods that must be cooked, like grains, meat, fish or dried beans, should be cooked as lightly and for as short a time as possible. This preserves their fiber, vitamins and some enzymes. Keep cooked dishes small and few and raw food dishes large and numerous.

- Follow the 80–10–10 formula. Combine your foods so that 80 per cent or more of your calories are derived from complex carbohydrates, a maximum of ten per cent from fats, and 10 per cent from protein.

- Eat twice as many vegetables as fruits. Vegetables are richer in chlorophyll, vitamins, minerals and fiber.

- Before eating any cooked dish, eat a large salad of fruits or vegetables first. Or eat a large amount of raw fruits or vegetables with the cooked item. This will supply some of the digestive enzymes, vitamins and fiber that have been destroyed by cooking.

- Avoid eating fruits and vegetables (and other incompatible combinations) at the same meal.

- Try to avoid all fatty foods except nuts, seeds and avocadoes.

- Get your protein from vegetarian sources or else from deep ocean fish, egg whites, very lean meat or very low-fat dairy foods.

- Eat as wide a variety of Restorative Foods as you can. Avoid eating the same foods every day.

We'll explain these guidelines as we go along. But first, I'm sure you'd like to know what a typical meal of Restorative Foods looks and tastes like.

Virginia W's Diet of Anti-Arthritic Wonder Foods

Let's see what Virginia W. is eating today. Virginia recovered from rheumatoid arthritis 7 years ago by replacing all Stressor and Allergy Foods with Restorative Foods. Here is her day's menu.

- **Breakfast: the fruit meal.** A mix of fresh, raw apples, bananas and pineapples. (Sometimes she adds coarse-cut oatmeal, lightly cooked.)
- **Lunch: the protein meal.** A large, raw vegetable platter consisting of lettuce, carrot, cucumber, soybean and mung bean sprouts, an ear of corn and an avocado. With it, Virginia ate 1½ ounces of mixed sunflower and sesame seeds and 1½ ounces of mixed, raw, unsalted nuts and peanuts.
- **Dinner: the starch meal.** A large raw vegetable platter consisting of lettuce, red cabbage, carrot, cauliflower, zucchini, rutabagas, alfalfa and wheat sprouts, and a whole tomato. With it, Virginia ate a potato and a sweet potato, both lightly baked.

To make digestion easier, Virginia tries to eat all fruits at one meal, all protein at another and all starches at a third meal each day. Within this framework, she eats different varieties of fruits, proteins and starches each day.

Natural Foods—
The Fast, Convenient Way to Eat

Except for grating up the rutabagas and peeling the avocado, cucumber and tomato (dipping in boiling water first), Virginia served each item whole. The entire meal occupied a wooden platter 12 × 24 inches. She did not spend any time chopping and mixing up a salad. She simply placed about 12 whole Romaine lettuce leaves on the platter along with a whole carrot, half a cucumber, an ear of corn and a handful of sprouts. The seeds and nuts were served in small bowls. She used a knife and fork to cut up the avocado and tomato, and a teaspoon to eat the nuts and seeds. The rest she simply picked up whole and bit into.

The breakfast fruit she peeled and chopped up immediately before eating and served in a bowl with a fork. Total serving and preparation time for each meal? From two to 8 minutes.

"There are no greasy dishes to wash," Virginia said. "No pots and pans to scrub out. No oven to clean and no cleansers to buy. I spend about five minutes a day watering and raising sprouts."

Fast, convenience foods? The type of Restorative Foods Virginia ate today took less time to prepare then most conventional fast foods and less time to clean up afterwards.

Instead of tearing down her health, as do commercial fast foods, Virginia's "fast, convenience" living foods gave her every nutrient her body needed to get better from arthritis and to stay well for life. Virginia remains at her optimum weight without paying any attention to calories, and she has not had a single flare-up in the entire 7 years.

Virginia did not need to add bran to her food because every single item was high in fiber. Every food supplied its own digestive enzymes. Every item was rich in vitamins and minerals. Virginia got all the protein, fat and carbohydrates her body required. And she didn't need to mask the taste with junk food sauce because she thoroughly enjoyed the rich mixture of taste nuances that each honest food provided.

Natural Foods End Most Digestive Problems for Good

Aren't uncooked foods difficult to digest?

Although some starchy foods, along with cereals and beans, are easier to digest cooked, most fruits, vegetables, nuts and seeds are easier to digest raw.

The reason is that raw foods carry their own enzymes which our bodies use in digesting the foods. For example, the enzyme protease is used in digesting protein, lipase in digesting fats, and amylase in digesting carbohydrates. Cooking depletes foods of enzymes needed for digestion.

Most people who experience gas or indigestion after eating raw foods are either overeating or they are combining foods the wrong way.

Vegetarians classify foods into four categories: vegetables, fruits, proteins and starches. Protein foods include nuts, beans and seeds (as well, of course, as all animal-derived foods). Starches include such starchy vegetables as yams, parsnips and potatoes. Almost all foods in any one category are compatible with one another. But the different categories should be combined only like this.

GOOD COMBINATIONS

- Vegetables and starchy foods
- Vegetables and protein foods

POOR COMBINATIONS

- Vegetables and fruits
- Proteins and fruits
- Starches and fruits
- Starches and proteins

Citrus fruits and melons often don't combine well with other foods and should be eaten alone.

Only Living Foods Contain Anti-Arthritic Nutrients

Only raw foods have any appreciable nutritional value because cooking, processing or storing destroys 50–70 per cent of most vitamins. For example, canning or freezing can destroy up to 90 per cent of a food's Vitamin B_6 value. Processed foods and frozen juices have lost almost all of their Vitamin C. Both B_6 and C are essential vitamins for reversing arthritis.

Cooking meats and vegetables destroys 85 per cent of most vitamins. The nutrients that most of us think exist in cooked and processed foods actually don't. Nutritional research is showing that modern processed foods often contain 66 per cent fewer vitamins than are listed for these foods in Government nutrition handbooks.

Living Foods End Both Colitis and Arthritis For Bernice W.

Bernice W. was 39 when she was diagnosed as suffering from ulcerative colitis. Her doctor placed her on a high-protein diet, high in saturated fats and low in fiber. Severe side effects prevented her doctor from using cortisone. But during the two following years, he prescribed no fewer than 14 different drugs, none of which produced the slightest benefit.

At age 42, Bernice was attacked by pains in her fingers, wrists and left knee. The pains appeared quite suddenly with stiffness and inflammation following. Her doctor diagnosed the new ailment as rheumatoid arthritis.

The two diseases combined turned Bernice into a bed-ridden invalid. Her colitis prevented Bernice from taking aspirin or any of the standard arthritis drugs. As a result, her doctor advised Bernice to have her colon removed and to move her bowels into a plastic bag hooked to her waist. She would then be able to take drugs for arthritis.

Bernice was shocked at the suggestion of a cure which would have turned her into a lifelong invalid. She turned to reading nutrition magazines. She learned of a Natural Hygiene health school located nearby, and the doctor in charge agreed to take her.

The Hygienic doctor was horrified at Bernice's condition and her diet of protein and drugs. He found she was also suffering from osteoporosis, bone loss brought on by the high-protein diet.

Although Bernice was slightly underweight, she was placed on a five day fast. All drugs were withheld. At the end of the fourth day with neither food nor drugs, Bernice became aware that the pains in her joints had almost disappeared. For the first time in months, she got out of bed and walked. Her constant diarrhea also ended during the fast.

She was placed on a diet of fresh, raw fruits, vegetables, nuts and seeds and told to stay with them for life. Bernice was amazed and delighted to watch both her colitis and arthritis gradually slip away. She took no more drugs. Within six weeks, she felt fully recovered.

Although doctors customarily place colitis patients on a diet of bland, cooked foods with lots of protein to "build up the body" Bernice experienced no difficulty at all in assimilating a diet of uncooked natural foods. The Hygienic doctor explained that this was because all living foods abound in enzymes needed for digestion.

All this took place 20 years ago. Now a fit and youthful 63, Bernice has remained a food "purist" and has had no trace of either colitis or arthritis. Except for lightly baking potatoes and other starchy vegetables, her diet consists exclusively of fresh, living foods.

How To Retain Nutrients While Cooking

To do the least harm to foods by cooking, cook as little as possible. Use as little water as you can, cook for the shortest time possible, and use the lowest temperature. Cooked foods should be crisp not waterlogged and soggy.

Light baking is probably the least damaging way to cook followed by steaming, cooking in a wok, or sautéeing with water instead of oil. Almost any type of starchy vegetable tastes delicious when lightly baked. Try to undercook as far as possible. Meat should be extremely rare.

Beans and cereals can be lightly cooked in a double cooker or crock pot. This way, you can minimize loss of vitamins, enzymes and fiber while cooking.

Boiling or stewing is least desirable because most vitamins are water soluble and dissolve in the cooking water. Frying, of course, is unthinkable.

You Can Continue to Eat Lots of Good Things

Bearing these principals in mind, there are still lots of good things you can continue to eat. Dozens of delicious, low-fat dishes can be made from corn, rice and other whole grains. Many Italian, oriental and other ethnic dishes are low in fat and can be safely prepared at home without salt or MSG. Whole grain spaghetti and other types of pasta are sold in health food stores and are superior to supermarket brands.

Tempting soups can be prepared from vegetables, beans or fruit and thickened with brown rice. For example, potato, cauliflower, onion, cabbage, tomato, celery, lentil, soybeans and white beans are all good in soups. Because you don't throw away the cooking water, soups retain more of their vitamins. Whole grain breads, pita bread and corn tortillas also go well with soups.

For sweet-tasting vegetables, try a mix of lightly-baked yams, parsnips and carrots with parsley. Adding onions, parsley, bay leaf and garlic to soups and cooked dishes adds spice to the taste. Parsley is rich in Vitamin A and other nutrients which arthritis sufferers often lack. To richen taste, blend foods with a mixture of raw tomatoes, cucumbers and avocados.

For a salad dressing, try one of the cold-pressed oils described later under Fats, or use a low-fat plain yogurt or cottage cheese.

You can eat eggs safely by simply hardboiling them, then removing the yolk and eating only the white. Or try a cholesterol-free omelette made of egg whites with sliced green onions and chopped parsley served on a slice of whole grain bread or toast. And, of course, literally scores of tasty dishes can be made by combining fish with vegetables and grains. Very lean meat and poultry can be alternated with fish for greater variety.

Desserts? Although it's wisest not to mix fruits with other types of foods, if you waited a short time after a meal, you could safely serve stewed prunes. Or a few dates and figs. Or a dish of fresh, mixed fruit. Or freeze a whole peeled banana and see if you can taste the difference between it and ice cream. Or freeze any fruit and put it through a juicer—it tastes delicious.

A Simple Eating Technique That Restores Enzymes and Fiber to Cooked Foods

You can overcome some of the drawbacks of cooked foods by eating a large salad of raw fruits or vegetables immediately before eating a cooked course. This gives you plenty of fiber and enzymes to work through your digestive tract ahead of the cooked course. Make sure the salad is substantial. Eat it all before starting on the cooked course. And finish the cooked course only if you are still hungry.

Len R. Overcomes Arthritis While Continuing to Eat the Cooked Foods He Loves

Len R. was a stocky former football player who loved "good food." By his mid-fifties, Len's love had added 60 surplus pounds to his already heavy frame, and he began to experience pain in his hips, knees and spine. His doctor said he had osteo-arthritis and advised him to lose weight.

Len went right on eating the cooked foods he loved. But his wife Celeste, who came from Switzerland, had other ideas. She re-read some old German treatises on Nature Cure that had belonged to her father. The books described a subtle way to prepare food for people who refuse to change their diet.

Celeste began making soups, stews, baked dishes and casseroles that tasted delicious but that were free of fats. And she preceded each meal with a raw vegetable salad. Len grumbled at the change in diet but admitted that the meals tasted good.

One morning, Len noticed that his pants seemed several inches too large around the waist. Lately, he'd also been feeling better. The pain in his joints had diminished. And he no longer needed laxatives.

Bit by bit, Celeste's salads grew larger and Len shed as much as 3 pounds per week. In a few months time his weight was back to normal and his arthritis pains had almost gone.

When Celeste explained it was all due to the change in diet, Len was finally convinced. He still continued to enjoy cooked foods. But by always eating a large salad first, Len transferred the benefits of living foods to the cooked foods he still loved.

Overcoming Arthritis the 80-10-10 Way

The 80-10-10 diet was developed for use at cardiac rehabilitation centers to reverse heart disease and hypertension. But recent reports from a number of university nutrition departments indicate it is also effective in reversing other degenerative diseases such as diabetes.

Essentially, the 80-10-10 formula means that 80 per cent of your calories are derived from complex carbohydrates, a maximum of ten per cent from fats, and ten per cent or so from protein. (Some nutritionists prefer that only 5 per cent should come from fats and 15 per cent from protein.)

What the 80-10-10 formula does is to ensure a diet low in fat and high in fiber with an adequate supply of protein and an abundance of natural vitamins, minerals and enzymes.

Although the 80-10-10 ratio is based on calorie content of food, if the total amount of your food consists 80 per cent of complex carbohydrates, 5–10 per cent fat, and 10–15 per cent protein you will be close enough.

Although nothing in this book urges you to go vegetarian,

should you decide to do so, increase the amount of protein-containing vegetarian foods to at least 35 per cent of the total quantity of food you eat.

Fat-Free Proteins That Restore Youthful Health

Protein should comprise 10–15 per cent of your diet. The one best source of whole protein for anyone with arthritis is deep ocean fish such as haddock or cod. Halibut, flounder and sole, and freshwater fish like mountain trout or catfish are also good if taken from unpolluted waters. Buy fresh fish if you can: the flesh should be firm, the eyes bright, the scales shiny and there should be a strong, fresh, briny smell. Frozen fish is next best. All oily or fatty fish or canned, smoked or dried fish, and all seafood and shellfish should be strictly avoided.

Once frozen fish is thawed, it must be eaten immediately. If you freeze your own fish, wrap them in moisture-vapor wrapping or glazing to prevent dehydration.

Cook fish with a low, gentle heat. Fish can be baked, broiled, sautéed or poached and made into a casserole. Almost all fish are rich in B-complex and other vitamins and in calcium, copper, iodine, iron, magnesium and phosphorous. Eat the bones if they are soft enough.

Other good low-fat sources of whole protein are chicken and turkey without the skin (the white flesh is best); lean beef, veal and other very lean meats; and very low-fat dairy foods like plain low-fat yogurt and cottage cheese. Baker's, Farmer's and Hoop cheeses are also low in fat and cholesterol. Egg whites are another cholesterol-free source of whole protein.

Although these foods are all low in fat and cholesterol, none contain any appreciable fiber or enzymes.

Proteins Without Cholesterol

If you are willing to take a little trouble, vegetarian protein is superior in every way. All vegetable protein is cholesterol-free, high in fiber, rich in enzymes and has an abundance of vitamins and minerals. Vegetable proteins are also less likely to be allergenic.

Good sources of vegetable protein are beans (especially

soybeans), nuts (especially pecans), peanuts, seeds, sprouts and grains. (Only the coconut is excluded because in the entire vegetable kingdom, it is the only food that contains cholesterol.)

No vegetable food contains all 8 Essential Amino Acids which the body needs to synthesize whole protein. To get all 8, you must eat a variety of protein-containing vegetarian foods all at the same meal once each day. Protein complementing, as it is known, is practiced by all vegetarians.

Harking back to Virginia W's protein lunch, it contained soybean and mung bean sprouts, an ear of corn, sunflower and sesame seeds, and mixed nuts and peanuts. The amino acids missing in one food were complemented by other amino acids in other foods to make up the necessary 8.

Fresh Garden Vegetables Without Soil

Sprouts are seldom if ever allergenic and are rich in protein, vitamins, minerals, enzymes and chlorophyll. Chlorophyll is the living green color in all leafy, green vegetables which transforms sunlight into energy. Chlorophyll could almost literally be called a "Miracle Food." A recent study at the University of Texas Systems Cancer Center in Houston identified chlorophyll as having powerful anti-cancer properties and it is a key nutrient in restoring health.

Almost all seeds, grains and beans can be sprouted. Alfalfa and mung beans, available at all health food stores, are easiest to begin with.

Simply place a half-inch depth of seeds in the bottom of a wide-mouth jar and soak in water overnight. Cover the mouth with cheesecloth or screen. Then rinse and drain 2–3 times a day. In 3–5 days, the jar will be filled with fresh, crunchy sprouts. Wheat and large seeds may take 7–10 days to grow. Eat wheat sprouts while they are about an inch long, otherwise they acquire a strong taste.

Most sprouts grow best in a warm room and in indirect sunlight. To turn them a rich green color, place them in full sunlight for the final day. This ensures they are rich in chlorophyll. Then store them in the refrigerator. Through sprouting, the original nutrient content of the seed is doubled or tripled. Sprouts are delicious in salads or sandwiches. They can also be lightly cooked.

Besides alfalfa and mung beans, you can sprout sunflower,

pumpkin, squash, mustard, lettuce, peas, sesame, wheat and many other seeds.

The Safe Way to Eat Fat

Our diets already contain too much fat for good health, hence the 80-10-10 formula seeks to restrict fat intake. What fat we need can be very adequately supplied by 3–4 ounces of nuts and seeds daily and a whole avocado. Fat from these sources is free of both cholesterol and rancidity.

In the unlikely event that more fat is needed, it can be obtained from cold-pressed, unrefined safflower, sunflower, soybean, cottonseed or corn oil. If you must fry foods, use one of these oils. The oil should not contain an oxident. Freshly squeezed, unsalted peanut butter is a safe food provided it is eaten promptly. By "freshly-squeezed" we mean squeezing it yourself a short time before use. Safflower oil mayonnaise sold in healthfood stores is considered a reasonably safe source of fat.

Shiela W's Arthritis Vanishes After Wonder Foods Sweep Out Her System

When Shiela W. was diagnosed as having rheumatoid arthritis, she was told to take 12 aspirins a day, to give up all exercise and to rest.

Instead, Shiela consulted a clinical ecologist—an allergist who specializes in foods. The ecologist put Shiela on a 5-day fast and found she was allergic to chicken, potatoes and cottage cheese. It turned out that Shiela was also addicted to these foods. At both breakfast and dinner, she would feast on baked chicken with baked potatoes smothered in cottage cheese.

Although Shiela firmly believed in nutritional therapy, she could not bring herself to give up the baked chicken, potatoes and cottage cheese. The ecologist tested Shiela's bowel transit time and found it took 4 days for this low-fiber food to pass through her system. The ecologist realized immediately that undigested particles of Shiela's addictive foods were passing into her bloodstream during their long, slow transit through her intestines.

Shiela was advised to eat a large, raw fruit salad before her regular breakfast and an equally large raw vegetable salad before her regular dinner. She was also to eat three thick slices of whole grain bread with her chicken at both breakfast and dinner. Another test a week later showed that Shiela's bowel transit time had been reduced to only 30 hours.

As the ecologist had guessed, the bulk and fiber in the raw salads and bread swept boldly through Shiela's intestines carrying the low-residue cooked chicken, potatoes and cottage cheese along with it.

As the time in which her undigested food particles spent in her intestines was cut, absorption of these foods into Shiela's bloodstream was also drastically reduced. This, in turn, cut the allergen reaction by Shiela's immune system and it stopped the auto-immune attack on her joints.

Eventually, Shiela was able to drop the addictive foods altogether and to replace them with nuts, seeds and avocadoes. In the 3 years since she took this step, she has stayed completely free of arthritis symptoms.

Complex Carbohydrates—
Nature's Miracle Anti-Arthritis Foods

Eighty per cent of all Restorative Foods should consist of fresh, living fruits, vegetables and grains. Because large amounts of fruit sugar can temporarily unbalance blood sugar levels, most nutritionists recommend eating at least twice as many vegetables and grains as fruits. This is why Virginia's menu featured two vegetable meals to one fruit meal. Also, vegetables supply a greater variety of vitamins and minerals.

Fruits, and particularly citrus, are good sources of Vitamin C, often called the "Arthritis Vitamin" because of its widespread role in arthritis recovery. So you need at least 4 fruits or fruit sections per day. If you eat more citrus, or use it for snacks, all well and good. Other fruits considered beneficial in arthritis recovery are bananas, apricots, berries and melons.

Try to avoid eating the skins of fruits that have been sprayed with pesticide. However, the skins of apples and similar fruits have such nutritional value that they should be eaten if at all possible. You can remove some of the pesticide residue by scrubbing fruit skins with a wire brush.

We'd also peel the skins of vegetables like cucumbers that may have been sprayed and then rubbed with oil by supermarket personnel. You can remove most of the pesticide residue from lettuce, celery and similar vegetables by removing the outer leaves or stalks and cutting off the top. This expedient is regrettable because many of the nutrients are contained in the skin.

The solution is to start your own organic garden and grow your own produce.

The Health-Promoting Properties of Certain Common Vegetables

All green, leafy vegetables are rich in chlorophyll. Tightly packed Iceberg lettuce is nutritionally inferior because the leaves are whitish and lacking in chlorophyll. Try to include plenty of yellow, red and darker colored vegetables in your salads and meals. Darker colored vegetables contain more nutrients.

Among food families, cruciferous vegetables are considered valuable in arthritis nutrition because they contain indoles, which inhibit the effect of toxins in the digestive tract. Also, the cruciferous family, which includes broccoli, cauliflower, Brussels sprouts and similar green, leafy vegetables, seldom causes allergies. Other vegetables often considered beneficial for arthritis nutrition are mushrooms, peas, soybeans, lima beans, tomatoes, carrots and avocados.

Most vegetables quickly lose their nutrients when they wilt. So pack them in plastic bags to keep them fresh longer. Try to avoid frozen vegetables.

Grains are the best sources of fiber and of B-vitamins. Coarse-cut oatmeal is a recommended breakfast cereal. It takes only a few minutes to cook in a double cooker. Serve with fruit or raisins.

Most packaged breakfast cereals have a high sugar content, granola among them. Among packaged cereals, shredded wheat and puffed rice seem lowest in sugar.

Bread made exclusively of whole grain flour and minus all eggs, fats, oils and sugar is a good health-restoring food. Yeast-free breads like unleavened bread and pita bread are less likely to be allergenic.

If you must have snacks, citrus fruits are best. Otherwise, chew on carrots, celery, sunflower seeds, nuts or apples.

The 80-10-10 Formula Galvanizes Jane R's Body into Throwing Off Arthritis

Jane R. was 45 when she was divorced. Soon afterwards, osteo-arthritis appeared in the joints of her fingers and toes. Pea-shaped knobs began to form on the end joints of her fingers, and her doctor diagnosed them as Heberden's Nodes. On each hand, the tips of her index and small fingers began to turn in towards the middle finger.

Her doctor's prognosis that nothing could be done sent Jane inquiring about alternative therapies. A friend who had had both hypertension and gout told Jane that, after changing his diet to overcome hypertension, the gout had also disappeared. The diet was the 80-10-10 formula which is often used by nutritionists in treating high blood pressure.

Under her friend's guidance, Jane changed over to a diet in which 80 per cent of her food consisted of fruits, vegetables and grains; ten per cent of nuts, seeds and avocados and ten per cent of fish and chicken.

Within a week, the 80-10-10 formula abruptly ended several minor ailments that had plagued Jane for years. Her chronic irregularity was replaced by easy, thrice-daily bowel movements. She no longer had frequent headaches. And her heartburn and acid stomach quickly disappeared.

Jane was so encouraged by these results that she stuck right with the 80-10-10 formula. Her roly-poly body gradually began to firm up, and in 8 weeks her figure was slim and trim.

At this point, she noticed that the pain and stiffness in her fingers and toes had disappeared. The disfiguring bony protuberances remained. But normal use of her fingers and toes had been completely restored.

Today, 5 years later, Jane continues to eat the 80-10-10 way. Her overall health has improved tremendously. She now plays tennis regularly and swims a mile nonstop 3 times each week. The only reminders of her bout with arthritis are the flat, spatulated joints at the ends of her fingers and toes.

Unusual Benefits from Unusual Beverages

For beverages, try some freshly-squeezed vegetable juices. They are preferable to fruit juices. Carrot juice goes particularly well with breakfast. You can juice vegetables in a blender. Carbonated spring water is a good substitute for soft drinks.

For a hot beverage, try carob or herb teas. Carob is a chocolate-like drink. Make sure the brand you buy is sugar-free.

An herbalist friend recommends the following teas as beneficial for arthritis: alfalfa, boneset, camomile, celery, linden, parsley, peppermint and wintergreen leaves. You can sweeten any hot drink with a little honey.

My herbalist friend particularly recommended Camomile Tea as a natural relaxant and sedative. She finds that it induces drowsiness and sleep and helps people with arthritis get a good night's sleep.

If your drinking water is heavily treated, or has tested allergy-positive, drink only bottled water.

Try to rotate all foods so they are eaten about 4 days apart. For example, you might eat walnuts one day, almonds the second day, Brazils the third day, and cashews the fourth day. It is not always possible to space out foods this far apart. But at least try to avoid eating a lot of any one food frequently. You *could* become addicted to such foods and they *could* become allergenic.

Eat Only Compatible Foods

Naturally, you would omit from your list of Restorative Foods any that you have tested out as allergy-positive. After an abstinence of several weeks, you may be able to eat some of them again at well-spaced-out intervals.

If you are living or eating with a family or group who continue to eat Stressor Foods, you must separate your food from theirs. You will need your own part of the refrigerator for fresh fruits and vegetables and you will find a bean crock and double cooker useful.

Easing Smoothly into Living Foods

Suppose you have an ailment which is aggravated by uncooked foods. In reality, very few ailments, including colitis, ulcers and gall bladder problems, are really irritated by uncooked foods.

If you do experience any digestive problems, make a

gradual transition from your present low-bulk, all-cooked diet to high-fiber Restorative Foods. Make the changeover gradually and in easy stages. Many people with digestive problems find it takes about six weeks to make the changeover. By that time, all their digestive problems have usually disappeared.

Naturally, if you are under medical care or taking medication for any ailment that might be affected by a change in diet, you should consult your doctor first.

Stay at the Peak of Good Health the Rest of Your Life

Be prepared to stay with Restorative Foods permanently. With a cyclical allergy you can cheat occasionally and get away with it. But people who stray back to fixed allergy foods often experience a flare-up of arthritis symptoms the following morning.

Whenever our health is at its highest peak, our resistance to arthritis is greatest. Fit, healthy people seldom if ever succumb to arthritis. An arthritis sufferer who attains the peak of health is able to shake off arthritis sooner.

Thus the obvious way to prevent or to reverse arthritis or gout is to live at the peak of good health all of the time.

CHAPTER 12

THE TEN
HEALTH-RENEWING POWERS
OF RESTORATIVE FOODS

Most professional healers in charge of arthritis clinics today consider that the disease is the result of nutritional deficiencies.

For example, Robert Bingham, M.D., Medical Director of the National Arthritis Medical Clinic at Desert Hot Springs, California, states: "It has been found that seven out of ten patients with arthritis will improve or recover after changes in their dietary habits. The type and quality of food intake of a patient with arthritis is extremely important. Most patients with arthritis have unrecognized dietary deficiencies and personal nutrition problems. Some patients lack essential items in their diet especially natural proteins, vitamins, minerals and enzymes. Some patients are underweight because of poor appetite, pain and the use of drugs. Others are overweight from consuming an excess of sugars and fats or from an inability to exercise because of joint pain and stiffness."

Osteo-arthritis, for instance, occurs when the bones, tissue and cartilage in a joint are weakened by nutritional deficiencies. At the same time, the nutritionally poor diet causes the victim to become overweight. When this excess weight is superimposed on the nutritionally weakened joint, the resulting wear and tear breaks down the bone, tissue and cartilage, creating the condition known as osteo-arthritis.

Osteo-arthritis can be turned around only by changing to a

diet of nutritionally-rich Restorative Foods. By restoring sound nutrition, the victim's weight gradually drops back to normal while the joint is also gradually able to restore itself from the abundant supply of essential nutrients available in the blood-stream.

How do Restorative Foods make good the various dietary deficiencies and other dysfunctions brought about by arthritis?

#1. By Restoring the Vitamin-Mineral-Enzyme Deficiency That Afflicts Almost Everyone with Arthritic Disease

Almost all men and women with any degree of severe arthritis have a serious deficiency of B-complex vitamins; Vitamins A, C, D, and E; and the minerals calcium, magnesium, manganese and zinc. Studies show that B-vitamin blood levels in persons with arthritis are as much as 75 per cent lower than in the general population. This routine deficiency depletes the body of many nutrients needed to keep the cells of joints, tissue, bone and muscle healthy.

For example, a deficiency of minerals like calcium, magnesium, manganese and zinc restricts production of synovial fluid, inhibiting lubrication in arthritic joints.

Deficiencies of Vitamin C and calcium have such serious effects that they must be considered separately.

Not only arthritis patients but almost all Americans 50 and over suffer from some degree of vitamin, mineral and enzyme deficiency. Partly this is because our modern, fat-laden animal foods nowadays contain significantly fewer nutrients than they did several decades ago when animals were leaner and healthier. Yet basic nutrition handbooks published by the Government continue to quote vitamin-mineral contents of animal foods based on research done decades ago.

For example, it was recently found that modern pork contains 30 per cent less iron than formerly while modern beef has 20 per cent less. Today's animals are simply fatter than in earlier times and the more fat in an animal, the fewer nutrients its tissues contain.

Again, refined foods are often enriched with supplements that are biologically unusable by the body. Also these foods that are enriched, like refined flour and milk, are high-risk Stressor Foods and should not be eaten anyway.

Restorative Foods Are Rich in Health-Building Nutrients

While millions of people do take vitamin and mineral supplements, here again many nutritionists believe these supplements are often biologically inactive and unusable. Before they can be utilized by the body, for instance, most mineral supplements must be in the form of complexes with amino acid or protein chelates. Single B vitamins like B_6 can produce benefits only when taken together with all other B-complex vitamins. And B_6 cannot be utilized unless zinc is present.

Again, calcium cannot be utilized unless adequate amounts of Vitamin D are present. Nor can calcium be utilized when the body's phosphorous level is high. Many Stressor Foods like meat and carbonated drinks have high levels of phosphorus and low levels of calcium. As a result, arthritis patients who eat large amounts of animal protein often have such low calcium levels that after several years, they lose their teeth and show a serious loss of skeletal bone.

Again, in a recent study published in the *Journal of the American Medical Association*, it was reported that zinc supplements could increase risk of heart attack by lowering the Lipoprotein fraction of cholesterol.

The requirements for proper absorption of vitamin and mineral supplements are often so exacting that most people are better off obtaining their vitamins and minerals from natural foods. Provided the foods are low in fat and high in fiber, the mix of vitamins and minerals is so varied that the right proportion of most nutrients is readily available.

Absorption difficulties, such as those some people encounter with milk, do not occur in Restorative Foods. In fruits, vegetables, nuts, seeds and grains, all minerals are naturally chelated, with absorption almost assured. And all of these living foods are rich in enzymes needed for digestion.

Dottie L. Discovers Amazing Benefits from Calcium-Rich Restorative Foods

"I was a heavy eater of sugar, white bread, pastries and junk food." This was 45-year old Dottie L. speaking. "By my fortieth birthday, I had pain and stiffness in my left knee, my neck and the wrists and fingers of both hands. Eventually I could hardly walk. My doctor diagnosed it as rheumatoid arthritis.

"The doctor told me to replace the refined foods with lots of meat, chicken and eggs and to cut out all dairy foods. This helped some. But my joints just became stiffer and bony overgrowths began to appear.

"It was obvious I wasn't getting any better. So I went to see a chiropractor who specializes in nutrition. He had me fast for five days, and I tested allergic to chicken, wheat, beef and yeast. I also took a hair mineral analysis that showed I was low in calcium, magnesium, manganese and zinc.

"I was advised to drop all high-protein foods and to eat only fresh fruits, grains and produce. The chiropractor said to eat plenty of low-fat yogurt and cruciferous vegetables to build up my calcium. I also took Vitamin D.

"Well, only fifteen days after the fast, my joint pains had almost disappeared. A month later I could walk and use my arms and wrists freely."

Gradually, the worst of the bony overgrowths broke up. Now, 3 years later, Dottie still has some disfigurement. But she remains free of pain as long as she stays with her diet, and she is more active than she has been since her teens.

#2. By Restoring Collagen Integrity

Arthritis has long been linked with collagen abnormality. Collagen, a body protein, comprises two thirds of all cartilage in our joints and it plays a vital role in the health of each joint and its supportive tissues.

The marginal nutrition supplied by Stressor Foods reduces the total amount of collagen in the connective tissues of each joint. Collagen breakdown is caused by insufficiency of Vitamins A, B_6 and C and the minerals magnesium and zinc. Vitamin C is absolutely essential in the formation and maintenance of collagen. Vitamin B_6, also essential for collagen production, must be taken daily together with other B-complex vitamins.

All of these nutrients are supplied in abundance by such Restorative Foods as fresh fruits, vegetables, nuts, seeds and whole grains.

Sound Nutrition Makes
Michael K.'s Heel Spur Disappear

A heel spur is a form of non-articular arthritis caused by a calcium deficiency. The condition begins with a minor injury typically caused by jogging on a hard concrete surface. The plantar fascia, a ligament extending from heel to toe, tears away from the heel bone. And a hard calcium spur grows in its place.

Like many doctors, Michael K.'s physician believed that his heel spur was due to a surplus of calcium in the body. So no diet change was recommended. Michael was fitted with orthotics (medically-designed heel lifts) and told to stop his daily jogging.

Michael began to go for long daily walks instead. But his heel became so painful he could scarcely bear to touch it to the ground.

A friend knowledgeable about nutrition recommended that Michael eat a head of Romaine lettuce every day with two cupfuls of low-fat cottage cheese as a dressing. Michael was also to sunbathe for 15 minutes daily.

Michael did as instructed. After several weeks, a strange thing happened. The pain in his heel gradually faded away. Exactly 8 weeks after he first began eating the lettuce and cottage cheese, and sunbathing each day, the pain in Michael's heel had disappeared.

Michael's friend instructed him to keep eating calcium-rich foods and to sunbathe regularly. Sunbathing, the friend explained, is Nature's way of ensuring an adequate supply of Vitamin D. During winter, when sunbathing became difficult, Michael took a daily capsule of Vitamin D.

Michael's recovery from a heel spur is just one of many similar instances I came across while talking with retired people around the country. In each case, recovery occurred when the person increased his or her intake of calcium and Vitamin D.

#3. By Improving Calcium Utilization

Although many doctors still believe that a surplus of calcium in the body causes deposits in arthritic joints, actually almost everyone with arthritic disease has a severe calcium deficiency. Whenever calcium levels in food and in the bloodstream are low, the parathyroid gland triggers release of calcium from skeletal bones, creating a condition of bone loss known as osteoporosis.

The calcium which is leached from bones and teeth is deposited in arthritic joints. This leaves the bones demineralized, fragile, brittle and easily broken. Osteoporosis is almost routine in middle-aged and older women with arthritis.

Osteoporosis begins with eating more animal protein than the body can handle. Studies have shown that women who eat large amounts of meat, eggs and poultry lose 35 per cent of their skeletal bone mass between ages 50 and 89, while vegetarian women lose only 18 per cent. These tests show that a high-protein diet doubles bone lose at any age.

Many nutritional studies have also proved that when a person with osteoporosis is placed on a low protein, high-complex carbohydrate diet rich in calcium and Vitamin D, bone density can gradually be rebuilt to normal. For example, a 1979 study at Kentucky State University found that when elderly women with osteoporosis were given a calcium-rich diet with Vitamin D, in six months time their bone density had increased by 25 per cent.

Restorative Foods rich in calcium include green leafy vegetables, whole grains, sesame and sunflower seeds, seaweeds, almonds, filberts, Brazil nuts and dried figs. But before it can utilize calcium, the body also needs Vitamin D. This vitamin can be obtained naturally by sunbathing for about 15 minutes daily. Or if that is not possible, it can be obtained by taking a daily Vitamin D supplement.

Ted C. Uses Restorative Foods to Overcome Severely Calcified Joints

Ever since high school, Ted C. had enjoyed running and weight lifting. He became so stocky and muscular that his upper body became a burden on his joints. At age 30, Ted's osteopath advised him to drop all foods containing calcium and to eat a high-protein diet.

Two years later, his spine, shoulders, knees and elbows were so stiff and painful, Ted had to give up pumping iron. X-rays revealed advanced osteo-arthritis and calcification in all joints. Ted was given Indocin and again told to eat lots of protein and to avoid calcium. But the calcium deposits became even worse. Spurs appeared on both heels and the osteopath said he would never run or lift weights again.

"At thirty-eight I had to give up all exercise," Ted said. "Finally, a friend who owned a health food store set me straight.

"He told me to cut down drastically on protein and to eat all the calcium-rich foods I could. I was also to take a daily supplement of Vitamin D. My friend said that the high-protein diet had caused calcium loss for years. My joints were filled with deposits of calcium leached from my bones and teeth. I was told to replace all the meat, eggs and chicken I'd been eating with a natural diet of fruits, vegetables, nuts, seeds and grains. And to stay with them for life."

The high protein foods that Ted now avoided included almost all types of Stressor Foods high in saturated fats. His new diet consisted entirely of Restorative Foods. Freed now from the excessive protein intake which had unbalanced his inner chemistry, Ted's body began to rebalance its calcium metabolism. Gradually, the pain in his joints disappeared. Ted lost no time in moving his joints again and breaking up the calcium deposits.

Four months after making his diet change, Ted was lifting weights once more. His heel spurs had disappeared and he was able to run again.

In the 8 years since, Ted has stayed rigidly with Restorative Foods. Throughout that time, his joints have stayed pain-free and flexible, and he has had no recurrence of arthritis symptoms.

#4. By Restoring the Deficiency of Vitamin C

According to a report in *Experientia* (vol. 35, No. 2, 1979) a Canadian research team recently cultured arthritic cells from a human joint afflicted with rheumatoid arthritis. It was found that these cells were sadly deficient in Vitamin C. When high levels of Vitamin C were given, the arthritic cells were eradicated while all normal cells continued to thrive.

Vitamin C, the chief custodian of collagen, is a powerful healer which is present in generous quantities in a healthy person's adrenal glands. But Vitamin C is so lacking in people with arthritic disease that, in a recent study at the Department of Pharmacology at Trinity College, Dublin, Ireland, it was found that 85 per cent of all people with rheumatoid arthritis were actually suffering from subclinical scurvy. The researchers found that Vitamin C is consumed faster in people with arthritis than in healthy people. One reason is that aspirin leaches Vitamin C from the blood. In doing so, it suppresses the immune system and lowers resistance to all infectious diseases.

Stressor Foods are particularly deficient in Vitamin C.

This lack of Vitamin C is believed responsible for causing the abnormality in the immune system that recognizes harmless food particles as foreign invaders. A deficiency of Vitamin C also leads to joint problems while an abundance of Vitamin C eases stress in joints.

By following the 80-10-10 formula, up to 80 per cent of a Restorative Food diet consists of fresh fruits and vegetables with ample nutritive ability to restore the deficiency of Vitamin C in the average arthritis patient.

#5. By Normalizing the Immune Response

Rheumatoid arthritis occurs when, through an abnormality, the white cells of the immune system identify food particles as foreign and then mistakenly attack the cells in our own joints. This abnormality does not occur in a totally healthy person with optimum nutrition.

Poor nutrition is a frequent cause of immune system suppression and abnormality. For example, research at such renowned institutions as Memorial Sloan-Kettering Cancer Center and the City of Hope National Medical Center in Duarte, California have demonstrated that performance of the immune system can be bolstered by an abundant supply of Vitamin C and zinc together with adequate amounts of Vitamin A and E and the B-complex. Several research scientists have hypothesized that this nutritional boost will also eliminate the abnormal reactions that lead to arthritis.

Restorative Foods rich in Vitamin C are leafy, green vegetables, citrus fruits, strawberries, broccoli, Brussels sprouts, tomatoes, turnip, cabbage, cantaloupe and honeydew melon, okra, potatoes and sweet red peppers. Zinc, a trace element, is present in many vegetables and grains. Carrots are rich in Vitamin A. And such foods as seeds, nuts, grains and leafy, green vegetables are good sources of B-complex vitamins.

Jack F. Ends Excruciating Gout with Health-Promoting Foods

At age 55, Jack F. had suffered from increasingly severe episodes of gout for over ten years. On his doctor's advice, Jack stopped eating foods containing purines. His attacks did become less frequent. But every few weeks, the joints in his feet and ankles would suddenly become hot, swollen, tender and throbbing, and the pain would last for several days.

Finally, a friend got Jack interested in nutrition. Although Jack had stopped eating foods containing purines, his diet still included large amounts of canned and cooked foods with almost no fresh fruits or produce. The friend advised Jack to cut out all foods that were refined, canned and processed and to replace them with natural foods containing Vitamin C. Jack was also advised to eat plenty of leafy, green vegetables, pecans, soybeans and brown rice for their B-complex vitamins.

At this writing, a full year has elapsed since Jack changed his diet. Throughout that time, he has not experienced a single gout attack. Recently, his doctor found that Jack's uric acid level had dropped back to normal.

The explanation? Jack's nutritionist friend believes that Vitamin C increases excretion of uric acid in the urine. But we must not forget, either, that Jack had also stopped eating most Stressor Foods and had replaced them with a diet of natural Restorative Foods. The chances are that, in doing so, he also removed the underlying cause of his gout.

#6. By Improving Elimination and Slowing Absorption of Toxins and Food Particles into the Bloodstream

No food of animal origin contains any fiber and all Stressor Foods are low-residue foods, meaning they pass slowly through the digestive system and are excreted in small, hard feces. Expelling these feces often causes straining and hemorrhoids. So it is hardly surprising to learn that almost all arthritis patients suffer from poor elimination.

On balance, Stressor Foods are so low in fiber (also called roughage or bulk) that they take 3–5 days to pass through the digestive system compared to less than a day for Restorative Foods.

This long transit time in the intestines allows far more undigested food particles to be absorbed into the bloodstream where they may set off the immune response and cause arthritis.

A long, slow transit time also gives bacteria in the intestines more time to break down decayed fecal matter and turn it into toxins that are also absorbed into the bloodstream. When this happens, other body organs such as the skin, lungs and kidneys are called on to eliminate the toxins. The breath becomes odorous, perspiration smells offensive, the skin is dry and rough, and the urine becomes dark and smelly. These signs of poor elimination are common in people with arthritis.

Nature's Cleansing Broom

These facts were medically confirmed by British researcher Dr. Dennis Burkitt and his colleagues while studying the effects of dietary fiber on colon cancer. They theorized that a high fiber diet protects against colon cancer by shortening the time food wastes take to pass through the digestive system. They found that in Africans living on natural, high-fiber diets, stools are so large and move through the intestines so rapidly that hazardous toxins are diluted and waste matter is quickly eliminated.

By comparison, the hard, sluggish stools of people in western industrial nations who consume large amounts of Stressor Foods pass so slowly through the intestines that bacteria are able to break down the natural bile acids and turn them into mutagens that cause colon cancer.

Writing in the *Journal of the American Medical Association* as far back as 1974, Dr. Burkitt stated his belief that lack of dietary fiber in refined foods and animal-derived foods is at least a partial cause of most degenerative diseases.

You can easily check your own transit time like this. After dinner, swallow some unchewed raw corn; or chew and swallow a whole cooked beet; or eat some blueberries. These markers will show up in the feces allowing you to check the exact length of transit time. The corn will appear exactly as you ate it; the beets will leave an unmistakable deep red color; and the blueberries will color the stool blue-green.

If your transit time is more than 36 hours, your diet is low in fiber. A diet of typical Restorative Foods will pass in from 15–30 hours with large, soft, unimpacted stools that sweep all toxins and waste matter clear out of the intestines.

Arthritis—The Cooked Food Disease

During a study in South Africa, it was found that while the bowel transit time for Europeans on a diet of low-residue foods averaged 90 hours, transit took only 18–24 hours for Africans on a raw diet of high-fiber foods. But when the Africans ate the same foods cooked, their transit time increased to 35 hours.

Cooking is another form of food processing that destroys all enzymes in all foods; it destroys the fiber in all foods but whole grains; it destroys some vitamins entirely; and many other vitamins and minerals are lost in cooking water. Because it destroys most fiber, cooking is also a major cause of constipation—a condition extremely common in people with gout or arthritis.

Just how detrimental cooking is to health was demonstrated in a classic experiment in 1946 by Dr. Francis Pottenger, an M.D. on the faculty of the University of California at Berkeley. Dr. Pottenger divided several hundred cats into two groups. One group was exclusively fed cooked meats and pasteurized milk while the other group got raw meat and raw milk.

Pottenger found that the group on the cooked diet developed a variety of food allergies along with arthritis and other degenerative diseases. Their immune systems were also suppressed to where they became susceptible to a variety of infections including pneumonia.

Dr. Pottenger found that the cooked food cats soon acquired the same ailments as humans eating the western industrialized diet. They became listless and fatigued. Many showed signs of diabetes, and as time went on, arthritis became widespread.

Many cooked food cats died while giving birth and their offspring were sickly and weak. Each generation showed more food allergies than the last. By the fourth generation, the cooked food cats were no longer able to reproduce.

Meanwhile, the raw food cats enjoyed optimum health and thrived.

Dr. Edward Howell, of Illinois and Florida, a pioneer researcher in enzymes, also found that cooked food passes through the colon more slowly than raw food. During the extended transit time, cooked food ferments causing gas, heartburn, headaches and colon diseases. Many colon specialists estimate that the average middle-aged meat-eating American is carrying a 3–4 day build up of waste fecal matter on his or her intestinal walls that weights from 8–30 pounds. This excess weight causes the colon to stretch and sag while toxic wastes seep into the bloodstream through the instestinal walls. During colonic irrigations, large quantities of hard, black fecal debris and cord-like mucous are expelled.

Both chronic constipation and diverticulosis can be permanently reversed in a few days by changing to a diet of Restorative Foods.

#7. By Normalizing Weight

The immediate cause of most cases of osteo-arthritis is wear and tear on joints caused by the burden of carrying surplus weight. When a changeover is made from a conventional diet of high-fat, low-fiber Stressor Foods to a low-fat, high-fiber diet of Restorative Foods, the total intake of calories is sharply reduced.

Studies of people who eat a high-fiber diet of Restorative Foods show that while such a diet is filling and satisfying, it is low in fat and calories. Indications are, also, that with an exclusively high-fiber diet, the body absorbs only those calories it actually needs from the digestive tract to maintain weight at its optimum level.

As Restorative Foods begin to rebalance body chemistry, one of the immediate results is to normalize the self-regulatory mechanism that controls appetite and weight through carbohydrate metabolism in the liver-pancreas system.

Recovering from osteo-arthritis through weight loss is covered in detail in Chapter 14. Persons with rheumatoid or similar forms of arthritis who have lost weight find that Restorative Foods will gradually rebuild their weight to the optimum level.

Restorative Foods Overcome a Severe Case of Osteo-Arthritis of the Spine

At age 55, Sarah D. had had osteo-arthritis of the spine for over 5 years. She was 30 pounds overweight. As a result of this excess poundage, arthritis symptoms were already appearing in her knees.

What made it all worse was Sarah's chronic constipation.

She rarely had a normal bowel movement. Once a week she would lie on the bathroom floor and give herself an enema. Afterwards, the toilet bowl was filled with hard, black fecal matter and stringy, cord-like excreta.

The explanation lay in Sarah's diet. She was inordinately fond of canned tunafish, salmon and sardines served on toasted white bread with potato chips and mayonnaise. Eggs, cheese, hamburger, hot dogs, pies, pastries, ice cream and coffee loomed large in the rest of her diet. She ate absolutely no fruits, vegetables, nuts, seeds or whole grains, and her intake of fiber was zero.

In the end, Sarah acquired the worst case of grapevine hemorrhoids her doctor had seen. Her stools were bloody and after each bowel movement, she had to push the hemorrhoids back inside her anus with her fingers.

Her sister had long been advising Sarah to change to a diet of natural foods. Sarah was so shaken by the hemorrhoids that she finally decided to take the plunge.

What her sister essentially advised was to give up all of the high-fat, low-fiber foods that are called Stressor Foods in this book and to replace them with a low-fat, high-fiber diet identical with our Restorative Foods.

Results were dramatic! Sarah's constipation, which had plagued her for half a lifetime, ended abruptly in just 48 hours. In place of the low-residue canned and refined foods that had taken a week to complete a bowel transit, the fiber-rich fruits, vegetables, grains, nuts and seeds she now ate swept lustily through her digestive system in a bare 24 hours.

Sarah no longer had to strain at stools. She went to the bathroom regularly every 8 hours. Her stools were bulky, soft and totally unimpacted.

Most astounding was the effect on Sarah herself. She felt better than she had in years. Without dieting or watching calories, her weight fell by two pounds each week and her spine and knees began to improve.

In 4 months, her weight was back to normal and her arthritis symptoms were fast disappearing. The hemorrhoids seemed better too.

Complete recovery took a full year. By that time, Sarah was able to walk several miles without pain or fatigue. She could bend her spine easily in all directions. And her hemorrhoids were no longer a problem.

#8. Through Boosting Production of
Natural Cortisone by the Adrenal Glands

All forms of arthritis are helped by increasing output of cortisone from the adrenal glands. Medical science capitalizes on this by injecting cortisone derivatives in the form of cortico-steroids (steroids) into joint tissue to suppress arthritic inflammation and pain. But when introduced artificially, cortisone throws the entire endocrine gland system out of balance, creating destructive and often life-threatening side effects.

Without going too deeply into the body chemistry involved, it has been found that foods rich in B-complex vitamins and Vitamin C can naturally stimulate the adrenal glands into releasing large amounts of cortisone.

Dr. C. E. Barton-Wright, a well-known rheumatologist, has speculated that both osteo- and rheumatoid arthritis are basically the result of a deficiency of Vitamins B_2 and B_6. These vitamins, together with Vitamin C, stimulate the pituitary gland to release the hormone ACTH which triggers the release of increased amounts of natural cortisone by the adrenals.

The cortisone-type hormones released by the adrenals diminish inflammation and destruction of cartilage in joints without any of the side effects of artificial hormones.

Restorative Foods like fruits, vegetables, nuts, seeds and grains contain ample supplies of Vitamin C and the B-complex vitamins to increase the output of adrenal cortisone.

#9. By Restoring Normal Blood
Circulation to Arthritic Joints

Atherosclerosis, or hardening of the arteries, is caused by a diet high in saturated fats and hydrogenated vegetable oils. Eating these stressful foods throws the body's self-regulatory systems off balance, leading to deposits of LDL cholesterol in arteries throughout the body. As these fatty deposits clog arteries and restrict the flow of blood, oxygen and essential nutrients to joints, the joints eventually become di-stressed.

Cardiac rehabilitation programs have proved that atherosclerosis can be reversed by a low-fat, low-protein diet high in fiber-rich complex carbohydrates. These restorative foods cleanse out the arteries and bring more blood and nutrients to inflamed joints and tissue.

#10. By Removing Toxic Flora from the Digestive Tract and Enhancing the Growth of Friendly Non-Toxic Bacteria

Saponin, a natural steroid found in certain plants, has a cleansing effect on the intestines which enhances the amount of enterocolic flora, a friendly organism, and which inhibits the growth of toxic micro-organisms.

Removal of these toxin-producing intestinal bacteria reduces toxicity in the bloodstream and in joints. As a result, saponin has a direct anti-inflammatory effect on enzymes in joints afflicted with rheumatoid arthritis.

The benefits of saponin were first revealed in a study reported in the *Journal of Applied Nutrition* (Vol. 27, No. 2 and 3, 1975) by rheumatologist Dr. Robert Bingham (an orthopedic surgeon and Medical Director of the National Arthritis Medical Center at Desert Hot Springs, California) and Dr. Bernard Bellew (physician and operator of an arthritic clinic in Desert Hot Springs, California). In the double-blind Bingham-Bellew study, 165 arthritis patients, ranging in age from 11 to 92, received supplements containing saponin and other nutrients obtained from a local desert plant or else they were given placebos.

Little effect was noted by those who received placebos, but 60.7 per cent of those receiving the saponin supplements reported significant relief of pain, swelling and stiffness. Reporting the study in the *Journal of Applied Nutrition*, Drs. Bingham and Bellew concluded: "In both osteo and rheumatoid forms of arthritis, (saponin) proved to have overall and specific beneficial effects."

In a similar study reportedly carried out by Dr. Robert A. Elliot of Woodland Hills, California, 50 per cent of patients reported noticeable relief after taking saponin-containing supplements. Another rheumatologist, Dr. Paul Isaacson of Tucson, Arizona, is also reported to have found that 50–90 per cent of his patients found some relief after taking saponin-containing tablets.

None of these doctors used saponin supplements alone. But all agreed that the saponin-containing supplements increased the success of other types of treatment also.

Saponin has been found to lower blood pressure, cholesterol and blood fat levels. It also appears to reduce frequency of migraine and asthma attacks. Some doctors speculate that saponin may reduce absorption of undigested food particles into the bloodstream, thereby reducing auto-immune attack on joints.

Saponin is nowadays readily available in health food stores. For instructions on how to use it, see under "Quick-Recovery Food #3" in Chapter 13.

CHAPTER 13

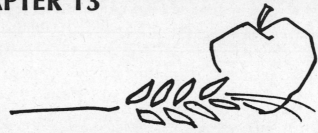

THE WONDERFUL ARTHRITIS-HEALING POWERS OF TEN QUICK-RECOVERY FOODS

When interviewed recently for a national periodical, Dr. Robert Bingham, Medical Director of the National Arthritis Medical Clinic in Desert Hot Springs, California, reportedly stated that a person with arthritis can significantly reduce pain and relieve stiffness and soreness in joints simply by eating foods containing essential vitamins, minerals and enzymes.

The vitamins and minerals known to reduce pain include Vitamins A, the B-complex, C, D, and E and the minerals calcium and magnesium.

Dr. Bingham's findings are being confirmed by modern science. As researchers are re-discovering the curative powers of plants and herbs, such modern drugs as digitalis are being produced from common plants. Drug companies have confirmed that herbs like comfrey are rich sources of vitamins, minerals and healing enzymes while others like yucca and alfalfa contain natural steroids.

Each of the ten Quick-Recovery Foods described in this chapter has a special bio-chemical application to joint cartilage. All are believed important in restoring the health of joint tissue. And all work Holistically to help reverse arthritis and gout.

Notwithstanding their undeniable therapeutic benefits,

you can find these commonplace foods on the shelves of almost every supermarket or health food store.

Eat them as snacks or as part of your meals. But because these foods act as a tonic doesn't necessarily mean that the more you eat, the greater the effect. Take them in moderate amounts. And eat only when hungry.

For these foods to work Holistically to reverse arthritis, the cause must be removed first. So all Stressor and Allergy Foods must be cut out before these foods can help restore your health.

If you know or suspect that you have one or more of the ten arthritis-linked deficiencies described in Chapter 12, by all means select one or more foods that you believe would help restore these conditions to normal. Then make them a regular part of your diet.

Naturally, you would not use any Quick-Recovery Foods to which you have tested allergy-positive. If you have any doubts as to whether you may have a sensitivity to any specific food, use the Quick Pulse Test (Chapter 8) to find out.

Although we don't recommend eating any food too often, or becoming addicted to it, most Quick-Recovery Foods are so nutritionally beneficial that they can be eaten daily during recovery from arthritic disease. After that, you might use all of them less frequently on a rotating basis.

Quick-Recovery Food #1: Boosting Intake of Certain Vitamins and Minerals Benefits Most Cases of Arthritis or Gout

Mollie R. first had rheumatoid arthritis at age 45. Treatment began with aspirin, but the pain in Mollie's hands and wrists became so intolerable that a few months later her doctor began using steroids. After three years on corticosteroids, Mollie's face had acquired a rounded, moon-like appearance, she felt constantly depressed and her condition had steadily deteriorated. Gradually, her knees and ankles also became targets for auto-immune attack. By age 49, Mollie could walk only with the aid of a cane. She consulted a second rheumatologist who urged surgery as the only alternative for her deteriorating left knee.

Finally, out of sheer frustration, Mollie went to a chiropractor who specialized in orthomolecular therapy. Instead of further drugs and surgery, the chiropractor ordered Mollie to eliminate all high-risk foods (our Stressor Foods) from her diet and to replace them with fresh fruits, vegetables, nuts and seeds (our Restorative Foods). He especially recommended a liberal serving of what he called the "Seeds and Citrus Mix."

To make it, mix a large handful of hulled sunflower seeds with two tablespoonfuls of unhulled sesame seeds. Sprinkle with sliced kelp or dulse (seaweed available in health food stores) and add two tablespoons of brewer's yeast. Then eat the whole thing together with a large grapefruit or with two oranges. On alternate days, you can eat it with a large tomato or with two or three smaller ones.

Mollie alternated a spoonful of the seeds with a mouthful of citrus or tomatoes. From the day she first began to eat the mix, Mollie never looked back. Along with her dietary change, she ceased taking all medication. The chiropractor also made her a heel lift that had her walking normally again within six weeks.

Rich in B-complex vitamins and Vitamins A, C, D, and E, the seed-citrus combination is also packed with calcium, magnesium, manganese, zinc and other anti-arthritic nutrients and enzymes. By her fiftieth birthday, Mollie was entirely free of all arthritic pain and stiffness.

In the five years since, she has had no serious arthritic flare-up, and each attack has been less severe and briefer than the previous one. She stays regularly with the "Seeds and Citrus Mix" which she thoroughly enjoys. And she finds that giving up the rich gremlin foods that she formerly ate was a small price to pay for her newfound freedom from pain and disablement.

Quick-Recovery Food #2: Five Years of Arthritic Pain Ends Abruptly When Herbert L. Switches to a Certain Breakfast Cereal

Soon after his fortieth birthday, Herbert L. was diagnosed as having rheumatoid arthritis of the right arm with degeneration of the spine. To kill the pain and reduce inflammation, his doctor prescribed 12 aspirins daily plus a periodic dosage of steroids. Herbert, who ran a plumbing business, often found the pain so intense that he took as many as 15 or even 20 aspirins daily. The aspirin caused severe stomach irritation. Yet nothing else helped.

That was until a knowledgeable aunt came to spend a vacation with Herbert and his wife. Although a self-taught amateur, the aunt was wise in the ways of nutrition. She was appalled by Herbert's diet, a seemingly endless round of rich meats, sausage, and cheeses with generous amounts of potato chips, white bread, cakes, pastries and sugary desserts, all washed down with gallons of coffee and soda drinks.

By her second day, the aunt had persuaded Herbert to make a radical change in the way he ate. So great was his discomfort that Herbert reluctantly agreed to try it. Because his aunt correctly diagnosed a severe deficiency in B-complex vitamins, Herbert was to begin each day with a cereal rich in Vitamins B_1, B_2, B_3, B_5 and B_6.

A Nutrient-Packed Arthritis Tonic That May Help End Pain for Good

For breakfast each morning, Herbert was to eat a bowl of cooked brown rice into which was mixed a large handful of wheat germ, two tablespoons of wheat bran and two tablespoons of brewer's yeast. Blackstrap molasses was added for sweetening. Atop the cereal and eaten along with it were numerous chunks of fresh pineapple and honeydew or cantaloupe melon. There was also a small side dish of pecans and sunflower seeds. Herbert nibbled at the nuts and seeds between spoonfuls of the cereal and fruit.

What Herbert was getting turned out to be two bowls of nutritional dynamite fairly bursting with thiamine (B_1), riboflavin (B_2), niacin (B_3), pantothenic acid (B_5) and pyridoxine (B_6) along with a generous supply of natural Vitamin C and enough fiber to thoroughly cleanse out his intestines and restore normal elimination.

Amazingly, Herbert began to feel better soon after his second breakfast with the new cereal. His aunt replaced the strong coffee with unlimited amounts of freshly-squeezed orange juice. She also urged Herbert to cease taking aspirin and any other drugs.

The pain Herbert dreaded never materialized. As the B-complex and C vitamins went to work to rebuild his collagen . . . to generate synovial fluid . . . and to stimulate his adrenal glands to produce more cortisone, Herbert felt increasingly cheerful and optimistic.

Although Herbert's pain and stiffness ended quite abruptly, complete recovery took considerably longer. But gradually, the symptoms tapered off and Herbert recovered full use and flexibility of his arm and back.

Herbert's speedy recovery should not surprise us. Tests have repeatedly shown that blood levels of B-complex and C vitamins in people with arthritis are often 75 per cent lower than in healthy men and women. When rheumatologist Dr. William Kaufman treated 663 arthritis patients with niacinamide (B_3), almost all reported gains in overcoming joint stiffness, muscle weakness and fatigue. More recently, Vitamin B_6 has also been found beneficial in relieving joint pain, especially in the hands.

More recently still, a combination of Vitamins C and B_6 (plus other B-complex vitamins) has been found to raise the threshold of immune response to allergenic foods. What this means is that an abundant supply of B-complex and C vitamins can reduce the pain and inflammation of rheumatoid and similar forms of arthritis caused by auto-immunity.

Quick-Recovery Food #3: Amazing Benefits from a Plant Extract Available at Any Health Food Store

Saponin, the naturally-occurring steroid hormone found in a desert plant called yucca, is readily available in tablet form at almost any health food store. When yucca extract tablets were given to 212 arthritis patients in a study by Drs. Laga, Harris and Bingham in California, approximately 66 per cent reported at least some benefit and relief from pain and swelling.

The tablets contained dry yucca juice, a natural medicine used by Indian tribes for hundreds of years to relieve arthritis pain. By taking from 2–8 tablets per day, the yucca extract produces an effect similar to cortisone on arthritis-caused inflammation. Yet yucca is entirely safe, natural and free of side effects.

For best results, you should take one tablet every four hours during the day (an average of 4 tablets daily). Larger, heavier people may take six or even eight tablets a day. Along with the yucca extract, you are advised to eat a liberal slice of avocado and a whole banana.

Alfalfa is another plant that also contains saponin. In tests, alfalfa has also lowered cholesterol and reduced headaches and arthritis pain. Alfalfa is best taken in the form of juice tablets sold in health food stores. Be sure not to confuse these tablets with others made from alfalfa leaves and stems.

You can boost intake of saponin by using a fairly strong brew of alfalfa tea as a beverage. To prepare it, stew one ounce of untreated alfalfa seeds (identical to those used for sprouting) in 2½ pints of water. Stir occasionally as it simmers for 30 minutes. Then strain out the seeds and drink up to 7 cups daily. Prepare a fresh brew every 24 hours.

Lorrie T. Uses Nature's Own Steroid to Reduce Her Swollen Joints

At 57, Lorrie T. had crippling rheumatoid arthritis pains in her hands and knees. She also suffered from diverticulosis and constipation so badly she could barely function. Her doctor had tried every type of medication but all Lorrie got was side effects.

On her 58th birthday, a friend advised Lorrie to change to a diet of natural foods and also to try taking yucca tablets. Exactly four days after starting, Lorrie began to go to the bathroom with unfailing regularity. A week later, her diverticulosis symptoms quietly faded away. Four weeks after that, her arthritis pains disappeared.

It took only another two months before Lorrie was up and about and moving as freely as she'd done 50 years before. At age 61, Lorrie now enjoys vigorous health and has had no hint of arthritis in the intervening 3 years.

Quick-Recovery Food #4: Nature's Own Analgesic Ends Pain from Rheumatoid Arthritis and Lumbago

Garlic, a common garden vegetable available in almost all supermarkets and in extract form at health food stores, contains selenium, a trace element which helps normalize the immune response.

When Japanese researchers tested garlic extract on patients with arthritis and lumbago, 86 per cent of the patients reported a noticeable improvement. None complained of side effects.

Dr. Satosi Kitahara, a Japanese professor of toxicology at Kumamoto University, has reportedly found that garlic extract aids in arthritis treatment by purifying the blood, removing toxins from cells and improving the circulation. Garlic's natural therapeutic qualities include beefing up the immune system, shedding surplus fat and rejuvenating the entire body.

Although you can and should add the natural garlic vegetable to any stew or similar dish when cooking, garlic extract capsules obtainable at most health food stores offer a more convenient and certain way to take garlic twice daily.

For best results, take one garlic capsule twice each day. The supplements are best taken along with a generous-sized helping of leafy-green lettuce and a fresh, ripe tomato.

Although garlic has been found most helpful for rheumatoid arthritis, it has also proved beneficial for both osteo-arthritis and gout. Be sure to take garlic supplements only in the form of capsule-enclosed oil. Dry powdered garlic is considered of lower value.

Quick-Recovery Food #5: Wonder Fruits That May Phase Out the Pain of Gouty Arthritis

A well-known Nature Cure clinic in the Southwest makes a point of serving half a pound of cherries twice daily to gout patients whenever the fruit is freshly available.

Their reasoning is based on the work of Dr. Ludwig N. Blair who, back in the 1940s, accidentally discovered that he could trigger a dramatic drop in his own blood uric acid level by eating half a pound or more of cherries each day. Although cherries are still the preferred fruit, subsequent experiments have shown that cherry juice is almost as effective. When neither is available, watercress and parsley are used followed in order of choice by cranberries, strawberries, pineapple and honeydew or cantaloupe melon.

Because research funds are available only for studies involving drugs, the specific nutrient factor in these fruits and vegetables that reduces uric acid has never been isolated. But since they are all rich in Vitamin C, cherries, watercress and parsley, cranberries, strawberries, pineapple and melons are also beneficial for all types of arthritis.

Unless organically grown, all berries should be thoroughly rinsed and washed to help remove any traces of pesticide before eating.

Whenever cherries are available, you may eat from ½–1 pound daily. Watercress and parsley can be liberally mixed in a fresh vegetable salad. When mixed with freshly-cut tomato, watercress also makes a tasty filling for whole grain pita or Arab bread. Alternatively, it can be used as a sandwich filling between two thin slices of whole grain bread. Other fruits can be eaten alone or mixed together in a tasty fruit salad.

Quick-Recovery Food #6: A Natural Health Booster That Renews and Recharges the Whole Body

Eight years ago, her doctor told Sue M. that she had a severe case of osteo-arthritis and that it would become increasingly worse with the passing of years. He told her to rest and relax, to avoid all vigorous activity and to take aspirin to relieve the pain and inflammation.

Sue did none of these things. Instead, she phoned the director of a well-known arthritis clinic in the Southwest and asked for his advice. Among the dietary changes suggested was a snack to be taken twice daily.

Each mid-morning and mid-afternoon, in place of her usual coffee break, Sue was to eat a large, fresh apple with an equal amount of fresh, raw carrot. The two were to be sliced up in a bowl and sprinkled with chopped kelp or dulse (seaweeds obtainable in healthfood stores).

Although her other dietary changes seemed beneficial, Sue felt most enthusaistic about the carrot-apple-seaweed snack. Each time she ate the snack, an hour or so later the stiffness and ache in her spine and knees became slightly less intense. Gradually, day by day, the arthritis symptoms subsided. Three months after she first began the twice-daily snack, Sue realized she was completely free of arthritis pain.

Although Sue has experienced an occasional return of pain since, each time it was briefer and less severe than before. Throughout the intervening eight years, Sue has not once missed her carrot-apple-seaweed snack. She plays tennis every day and is able to run, walk, swim or ride a bicycle with ease.

To prepare the snack, rinse and scrub the apple well before serving if it is not organic. But under no circumstances peel the apple. Apple skins are rich in pectin, one of Nature's most effective dietary cleansing agents. Tests have shown that pectin "scrubs" cholesterol out of the arteries and keeps blood vessels youthful and flexible. Pectin also moistens and helps eliminate any hard, dry feces in the colon.

Raw carrots are rich in calcium, magnesium, manganese and Vitamin A and help normalize the self-regulatory action of the liver-pancreas systems. Carrots also exert a profound and lasting improvement in elimination and colon action. In a study reported in the *American Journal of Clinical Nutrition* (September 1979) when researchers at the Western General Hospital in Edinburgh, Scotland fed 7 ounces of raw carrots to 5 healthy people each day for 3 weeks, their blood cholesterol levels dropped by 11 per cent. Their stool weights also increased by 25 per cent while bile acid excretion in the stools rose by 50 per cent.

Quick-Recovery Food #7: A Mineral-Rich
Natural Oil Helps Carole R.
Phase Out Years of Arthritis Pain

The story of Carole R.'s rheumatoid arthritis reads like a textbook case history. It began with a small swelling in the middle joint of her right index finger. Soon, the entire finger became swollen. Carole could not bend it. Three months later, all the fingers of her right hand were painful and swollen. Pain appeared next in her ankles, neck, shoulders, wrists and elbows. As she got out of bed each morning, the aching and stiffness in these joints was almost unbearable.

Carole's doctor gave her the usual X-rays and tests for rheumatoid factor, uric acid level, sedimentation rate, blood count and urinalysis. When the results came in, Carole was given the standard textbook verdict: "You have a severe case of rheumatoid arthritis. There is no known cure. Take plenty of rest and relaxation. Avoid strenuous activity. Eat plenty of protein. And take aspirin to relieve the tenderness and inflammation."

Just as medical textbooks predict, Carole began a life of crippling pain, disablement and deformity that was to last for three further agony-filled years.

That it did not last longer was entirely due to the arrival in Carole's town of a doctor of naturopathy who had been trained at a Nature Cure clinic that specialized in arthritis. Completely disenchanted by now with medicine's failure to relieve her suffering, Carole made an appointment with the naturopath on the first day that he opened his office.

The naturopath diagnosed Carole as suffering from faulty calcium metabolism. Her Vitamin D intake was so low that her body was unable to absorb the calcium in her food. As a result, calcium was being leached out of her bones and teeth and forming into deposits that restricted movement in her afflicted joints.

Among the naturopath's advice was a recommendation to take a tablespoon of cod liver oil twice each day. The naturopath explained that this natural fish oil supplies biologically active Vitamin D that is needed before the body can utilize calcium in food.

Cod liver oil is also rich in Vitamin A which is believed to help normalize immune system function and to stimulate regeneration of damaged tissue.

For several weeks, Carole noticed no difference. Then one morning, she detected a new flexibility in her normally stiff right elbow.

The following morning, the fingers of her right hand seemed more mobile than usual. Day by day, the stiffness slowly faded from her joints. Once she could move her joints without pain, Carole could feel the calcium deposits cracking and creaking. To help the deposits break up, the naturopath advised Carole to do lots of easy stretching and bending movements.

This therapy was so effective that 3 months after first taking cod liver oil, Carole was able to walk normally and to swing her arms freely over her head.

In the intervening 4 years, during which Carole has never once missed her ration of cod liver oil, her condition has constantly improved. Today, her bone density is completely normal and she has no trace of either arthritis or osteoporosis (skeletal bone loss).

Quick-Recovery Food #8: How a Condiment and a Sweetener Made Arthritis a Memory for Eva C

Eva C., a former schoolteacher, had suffered with rheumatoid arthritis on and off for over ten years. At times, she experienced a spontaneous remission. But often on winter evenings, she could barely move her elbows and wrists.

One day, a neighbor who had grown up in rural New England recalled that her grandparents had often taken honey and vinegar to relieve their arthritis. More recent investigation suggests that the acid present in apple cider vinegar does help to dissolve calcium deposits in afflicted joints.

Eva C. was instructed to take two teaspoonfuls of apple cider vinegar together with the same amount of honey in a glass of water at each meal. She was also advised to use apple cider vinegar liberally as a salad dressing and condiment.

Folk remedy or not, Eva's pain gradually vanished. The swelling in her wrists and elbows has subsided. During the 3 year period since she first began to take the honey and vinegar, she has experienced an occasional flare-up of arthritis symptoms. But each recurrence has been briefer and milder than the one before. Eva can now use both arms freely and has been almost completely free of pain for 36 months.

Quick-Recovery Food #9: Dramatic Results from a Gentle Curative Agent

During the late 1970s, the U.S. Department of Agriculture made a study in which several different types of animals were raised on a diet rich in yogurt. Results revealed that all the animals fed yogurt grew larger, stronger and healthier than comparable control animals fed a normal diet. Similar studies on both animals and humans have prompted many biologists to believe that yogurt contains an unidentified nutrient that promotes health and well-being.

Despite its containing cholesterol, yogurt actually lowers the serum cholesterol level when eaten regularly. Its calcium and acid content have also proved extremely beneficial in numerous cases of gouty arthritis.

To be of therapeutic value, yogurt must contain lactobacillus acidolphilus—a micro-organism that has demonstrated powerful antibiotic properties against unfriendly bacteria that afflict the intestinal tract. As a result, acidolphilus yogurt has special properties for restoring health during recovery from arthritic disease.

Not all commercial yogurts contain acidolphilus but most health food stores carry brands that do. Or you can easily make your own yogurt with acidophilus starter.

A Substitute If You Cannot Tolerate Milk

Researchers believe that fermented foods like yogurt can be tolerated by many people with a food sensitivity to milk. Yogurt bacteria apparently digest some of the lactose or sugar in milk, thus transforming it into a non-allergenic food.

During the same USDS studies, when control rats were fed equal amounts of milk fortified with massive doses of vitamins, the yogurt-fed rats still outperformed them.

One arthritis clinic has experimented with yogurt as a restorative food and found encouraging results. The recommended amount is 16 ounces of plain, low-fat acidolphilus yogurt divided into 3 portions and served as a snack 3 times daily. (That is, a full pound is eaten each day.) The yogurt must be free of any additional sugar, gelatin, flavoring or additives. If preferred, a small amount of honey may be used for flavor. Or, as in the Balkans, yogurt can be eaten with whole grain bread.

Observations have shown that this Restorative Food is even more effective when combined with 15 minutes of daily sunbathing. Sunbathing is Nature's way of providing Vitamin D. (If this is not possible, consider taking two tablespoons of cod liver oil daily or the same amount in capsule form.)

Walter W., a patient at the arthritis clinic, had suffered with severe gout symptoms in his hands, feet and knees during each of the previous 5 winters. During January and February each year, his uric acid level was as high as 13 mg/dl.

After spending the month of September at the clinic and becoming accustomed to eating the yogurt snack 3 times each day on a permanent basis, Walter was completely free of gout throughout the following winter. He has since continued to take the yogurt snacks regularly every day and has had no recurrence of gout at any time during the succeeding 5 years.

Quick-Recovery Food #10: Why the
Seaweed-Eating Japanese Seldom Got Gout

Until the mid-1960s gout was almost unknown among working class Japanese. For decades preceding the early 1960s, the average Japanese lived largely on soybean curd, fish, seaweed and brown rice.

Then came a new affluence that changed the diet of even the poorest classes. Nowadays, brown rice is considered "peasant food." This nutrient-rich whole grain has been replaced by denatured polished rice which contains little else but empty calories. Along with the new affluence has come white flour (called "American flour"), deep fried foods, rich meats and a variety of pickled junk foods, sugar drinks and candy.

Not surprisingly, by the early 1970s, Japan experienced a skyrocketing surge in almost every degenerative disease including not only gout and arthritis but heart disease, cancer, diabetes and hypertension. Previously, when most Japanese had lived on a low-fat diet of natural, largely high-fiber foods, these diseases had been approximately one tenth as common as in the U.S.

A Medicinal Diet for Arthritic Disease

Many nutritionists believe that it was their diet of brown rice, bean curd and seaweed that kept the Japanese almost entirely free of gout in earlier times. This belief has spread to several arthritis clinics and health resorts in Europe where brown rice is used as a medicinal diet in treating heart disease, hypertension, gout and arthritis.

But you don't need to visit a European spa to include brown rice, seaweed and bean curd in your diet. Brown rice, preferably organically grown, is widely available in almost every health food store and granary along with seaweeds from Japan. Alternatively, you may use less expensive American seaweeds like kelp or dulse.

Tofu, a cheese-like curd made from soybeans, is also now available in most larger supermarkets and health food stores.

To enjoy the same beneficial diet that the Japanese once had, build two or three meals weekly around a liberal helping of brown rice prepared in a double cooker or in a slow bean crock. Add nothing to the rice but water. Atop the rice serve an assortment of lightly-steamed vegetables including Vitamin-C rich Brussels sprouts, broccoli, turnips, cabbage, pineapple and seaweed, all flavored with garlic. If you prefer, you may prepare the vegetables in a wok.

Some people prefer to cook the tofu along with the vegetables. But we have found it better to add the tofu after cooking. Alternatively, also, you may sprinkle chopped seaweed on the vegetables after cooking.

For anyone who tests allergic to corn, oats, potatoes or other staples, brown rice is a wonderful anti-arthritic alternative.

CHAPTER 14

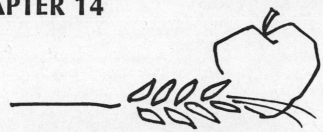

BEATING ARTHRITIS
AND GOUT WITH
FAT-DESTROYING FOODS

Statistics show that most people with gout or osteo-arthritis are overweight. Surplus poundage is usually the reason why osteo-arthritis occurs. Excessive body weight simply overburdens the weight-bearing joints in the spine, hips and knees. Under the stress of this continual weight, the protective cartilage in the joint loses its elasticity and wears away, exposing the bones in the joint to grate painfully against each other.

Cartilage breaks down under excessive weight only when it is deficient in essential nutrients. Nutritional deficiency is almost standard in anyone who lives on a diet of Stressor Foods. Stressor Foods are also responsible for excessive weight. So Stressor Foods are the basic cause of osteo-arthritis.

Gout is a disease caused by frequent indulgence in foods rich in purines (the basic component of uric acid). Purine-rich foods are all high in fat. Hence people who eat them soon become overweight.

Once pain and inability to move appear, victims of both diseases are less likely to keep their weight down by activity and movement. And since many doctors still believe that diet has no effect on arthritic disease, patients are often not advised to change their diet and lose weight.

Yet both diseases are directly caused by food. And both diseases can be greatly benefitted by a change in eating habits that leads to weight loss. In fact, records show that for symptoms to completely disappear, a patient must restore his or her weight to normal.

In case you're thinking in terms of a fad diet, relax! Seldom do any of the crash diets you read about lead to permanent weight reduction. The safe, natural way to shed surplus pounds, and to keep them off for good, has already been described in this book.

It simply amounts to eating only Restorative Foods and eating them the 80-10-10 way.

Losing Weight While You Continue to Eat All You Want

How can eating lead to weight loss?

Because Restorative Foods are all low in fats and calories and high in enzymes and fiber. Living foods like fresh fruits and vegetables all contain enzymes which activate fat loss in cells and aid in excreting fats and toxins from the body. These enzymes also help prevent fats and sugars in food from turning into fat deposits when eaten.

Among the many doctors who have praised the benefits of low fat, high-fiber natural foods is Dr. Neil Solomon. While recently on the staff of Johns Hopkins Hospital, Baltimore, Dr. Solomon reportedly said that most metabolic disorders can be reversed with a low calorie diet. Virtually all degenerative diseases are metabolic disorders and, as nutritionists have discovered, many can be permanently reversed by changing to a diet of Restorative Foods.

So powerful are the effects of a diet low in calories and high in fiber that many vegetarians are able to eat 4,000 or more calories daily without ever adding weight. Several studies have shown that when at least 80 per cent of the diet consists of fresh, uncooked fruits and vegetables, the fiber content is so high that the body will absorb only the calories it actually needs and will allow the remainder to pass through the intestines unused.

Fat-Destroying Foods

This means that a diet of fresh fruits and vegetables with whole grains is the most effective way to restore normal weight.

Provided you follow the 80-10-10 formula, you can eat all the Restorative Foods you wish without counting calories.

If you are overweight, you will gradually lose weight. If underweight, you will gradually gain weight.

To ensure a natural, healthful return to your optimum weight, 80 per cent of your diet must consist of complex carbohydrates; 5–10 per cent can consist of fat; and 10–15 per cent of complete protein. For more rapid weight loss, I suggest avoiding nuts, seeds and avocados and replacing them with protein-rich soybeans and other beans, both sprouted and cooked. As soon as your weight normalizes, you can go back to nuts, seeds and avocados.

Adding bran to conventional food does increase fiber and improve regularity. But it does not ensure weight loss. By contrast, a diet that consists exclusively of high-fiber foods requires extensive chewing. You will feel full and satisfied long before you can overeat. By eating Restorative Foods the 80-10-10 way, your food is so bulky you seldom feel hungry.

To shed weight, all you need do is to follow the nutritional therapy described in this book for recovery from arthritis. By cutting out all Stressor Foods, you eliminate most foods high in fat. And by undertaking a 5-day fast, you can lose as much as 8–10 pounds right away.

Shed Fat While The Body Purifies Itself

Fasting is the most rapid way to melt off pounds. While fasting, excess feces are removed and the intestines cleaned out while the body feeds off its own fat cells.

Before fasting, be sure to study Chapter 5 in detail, especially the section entitled, "Who Should Not Undertake the Purifying Technique."

If you are under medical treatment for any condition that might be affected by fasting or a change in diet, you should consult your doctor first.

Therapeutic fasting was pioneered and developed in America by practitioners of the Natural Hygiene movement (Natural Health Science). Their rules for safe fasting is that no one should fast for more than 5 days without professional supervision nor should anyone fast on their own for more than ten days in any one month period.

Staying within these guidelines, you could still fast on your own for 5 days every two weeks, alternating with Restorative Foods in between. You would typically fast for 5 days, then break the fast and return to eating Restorative Foods the 80-10-10 way for the following ten days. You could repeat this cycle indefinitely until your weight returned to normal.

By following this Alternate-Eating Program, most overweight people should be able to lose at least half a pound per day safely and naturally.

Through alternatively eating and fasting, your taste buds are tuned in to the new wavelengths of Restorative Foods. After a few weeks of living foods, most people are turned off by sweet, sugary junk foods and foods high in fat. As long as you continue to eat Restorative Foods the 80-10-10 way, the surplus weight will never return.

Anna J. Shrinks Away Fat and Loses Her Arthritis

According to standard height-weight tables, Anna J. should have weighed 130 pounds. But at age 55 she actually weighed 180. The burden of carrying around this surplus poundage caused such di-stress in her knees and hips that severe osteo-arthritis set in. Gradually, the pain spread into her upper spine, and her shoulders became almost too stiff to move.

Anna knew that losing weight was her only hope. But she was simply unable to count calories or to diet.

One morning, she woke to find the pain in her hips had spread into her groin and down the insides of her thighs. She could barely shuffle around the house.

"It was just too much," Anna said. "That was my moment of truth. I decided then and there that I was going to take charge of my body and I was going to get well."

Anna enrolled at a Natural Hygiene health school in the next state. The Hygienic doctor was aghast at her diet. Almost all of Anna's meals consisted of sugar and fat.

Anna was placed on an Alternate-Eating Program. This meant fasting for 5 days followed by ten days of fresh, raw fruits and vegetables.

In a single month, Anna had lost 20 pounds and she felt

sufficiently confident to continue the program at home. Another month of the program brought her weight down to 140.

As the pounds melted away, Anna felt better every day. The pain in her thighs and groin had disappeared. She could move her spine and shoulders freely again. And discomfort was steadily diminishing in her knees and hips.

Anna lost her last ten pounds on Restorative Foods alone. As the final pounds disappeared, she was able to do housework again and she began taking daily walks.

"I had to buy an entire new wardrobe," she said. "I went down from a size eighteen and a half to a size twelve."

That was 5 years ago. Anna still has the same trim figure and she is totally active and fit. How has she managed to stay on Restorative Foods?

"At the Hygienic School I learned that only fruits, vegetables, nuts and seeds are compatible with the human digestive system. Milk is all right for calves and beef for predatory animals like dogs or cats. But man cannot eat refined foods or foods high in fats without eventually becoming sick.

"Now that I'm well, I intend to stay that way. As far as I'm concerned, any kind of processed or fatty food is not fit for human consumption. I wouldn't eat any of those junker foods for a million dollars."

Miracle Eating Techniques That Melt Fat Away

Fasting for 5 days usually means taking time off from work. If this isn't convenient, ask your health food store proprietor for a protein supplement. By eating only protein, most people can continue to lose weight without experiencing weakness or hunger. Even with a protein supplement, you should not fast for more than 5 days without professional supervision.

Another natural alternative is a juice fast. This allows you to drink unlimited amounts of freshly-squeezed fruit or vegetable juices (plus all the pure water you need). In reality, a juice fast is simply a very low-fat diet. Provided you feel fit and energetic, it is possible to continue a juice fast beyond 5 days. But since it has no fiber or protein, it should not be continued indefinitely.

Juices can be made with a blender. Avoid canned juices.

Never mix fruit and vegetable juices. Try to drink more vegetable than fruit juice. Fruit juice should be cut with an equal amount of water to prevent a sudden flush of sugar into the bloodstream. Good vegetables for juicing are carrots, celery, cucumbers, Swiss chard and tomatoes.

Yet another quick weight-loss alternative is the mono-fruit diet. This allows you to eat all you want of any one fruit such as watermelon, grapes, apple or papaya. But you take nothing else except pure water. The fruit provides adequate energy and some fiber but no fat or protein. It should not be continued indefinitely.

Both the fruit juice fast and the mono-fruit diet aid in self-purification and give the intestines a thorough cleansing.

Jacob R. Eats Away His Gout with Fat-Destroying Foods

Jacob R. had suffered from periodic attacks of gout for more than ten years. His doctor prescribed drugs to lower his uric acid level and to dissolve uric acid crystals in his joints. But the drugs caused severe nausea, diarrhea and stomach distress.

A native of Germany, Jacob was well aware that gout was caused by foods high in purines and by his 40 pounds of excess weight. Jacob was also familiar with weight-loss methods used in European health spas. At the time he had left Germany 35 years earlier, the most popular method had been the mono-fruit diet.

Whenever Jacob had to stop taking medication due to severe side effects, the intense throbbing pain of gout would reappear in his feet.

"Finally, I told myself I'd had enough," is how Jacob himself put it. "It wasn't the drugs. I'd brought it all on myself by unwise eating. Right then and there I decided to clean up my nutrition.

"Watermelon was cheap at the time. So I started on a mono-fruit diet of watermelon. I could eat watermelon in unlimited amounts. But nothing else. No beverages. Nothing to drink, but all the pure water I needed.

"I knew that eating a single fruit would make minimum demands on my digestive system. It's the next best thing to fasting. But the watermelon gave me enough energy to keep on at my job.

"I stuck with the watermelon for four weeks and I lost twenty pounds. My gout didn't improve, though. It actually got worse. But I wasn't alarmed. I knew this was because, as my fat cells broke down, they released uric acid that had been stored up for years."

Jacob then resorted to what he called a "Nature Cure" diet which is virtually identical with our Restorative Foods.

"I left out all nuts, seeds and avocadoes though until my weight had dropped back all the way to normal," he told me. "Towards the end, my gout pains became less frequent. As I lost the final five pounds, they just faded away. And I've not had another flare-up since."

That's because Jacob has stayed strictly with his "Nature Cure" diet for an entire decade. Lean, fit and suntanned at 70, Jacob fairly radiates glowing good health. Five mornings each week he conducts an exercise class at the retirement community where he lives, and he is widely known as a natural foods enthusiast.

An Eating Technique That Shrinks Your Waistline

End any type of fasting or alternative-eating program whenever your ideal weight is reached. Your ideal weight is that shown in standard life-insurance height-weight tables. There is no health advantage in dropping below the recommended weight for your height.

You can prevent much weight gain by eating earlier in the day. The U.S. Army Research and Development Command recently discovered that the earlier in the day you eat, the less fat you are likely to gain.

The explanation? Calories eaten before 11 a.m. are burned up during the day before they can turn into fat. But calories eaten later in the day, especially in the evening, turn into fat overnight.

To capitalize on this phenomenon, eat your largest and heaviest meal for breakfast and schedule it early—as soon as you get up if possible. Make lunch your second heaviest meal and schedule it, too, as early as possible. Then eat lightly through the rest of the day.

Weight-loss can be speeded up still more by using the mini-meal routine described in Chapter 15.

How to Stop Using Food for Solace

Are you one of those people who eat too much because of what is eating you? If so, whenever you head for the refrigerator, stop and ask yourself why you are about to eat. Are you using food to smoothe the stress of anxiety, boredom, loneliness, or feeling unhappy, unwanted and unloved?

The solution here is to make a list of alternative pleasures, each of which is readily available and easy to do. For example, you might make love, listen to music, take a drive, go fishing, paint a picture, see a movie, read a novel or do something physically active if you are able.

Whenever you feel the urge to eat, sample an alternative pleasure instead. Try to disassociate eating with pleasures like drinking, reading or listening to music or watching TV or a movie. Never eat during these activities. Make eating an entirely separate activity.

For months following her divorce, Georgia R. would head for the refrigerator and load up on ice cream, pie, cookies and sodas. Georgia's inevitable gain in weight finally brought on osteo-arthritis in her knees. A psychologist friend suggested she find a substitute pleasure that brought more solace than compulsive eating.

Georgia had always wanted to paint. So she bought materials and took lessons in watercolor. Whenever she gets a downer, instead of heading for the refrigerator, she takes her easel and starts to paint. This motivational therapy worked so well for Georgia that over a 12 months period, her weight gradually dropped back to normal and her knees are pain-free once more.

Enjoy Life and Stay Thin

This might be a good place to mention the powerful benefits of movement and activity.

Once you have recovered sufficiently to move freely without pain, you should begin regular activity that involves gentle and easy yet progressive movements. The bending and stretching positions of yoga and the gentle, flowing movements of Tai Chi (a form of oriental martial arts) are perfect for breaking up calcium deposits and restoring flexibility to once afflicted joints.

As recovery progresses, begin regular daily walks and such enjoyable activities as dancing, bicycling or swimming. Many of the people in our case histories took immediate advantage of their ability to move again by becoming very active. Activity boosts the health-restoring powers of nutrition and helps maintain the entire organism in optimum health. It also prevents weight gain.

So use your body to enjoy life and to keep your weight down. Dance, play tennis or golf (without a cart), go canoeing or for bicycle rides, grow your own fruits and vegetables or join an adult fitness club. Once you take up the active life, it's next to impossible to put on weight again or to get arthritis.

CHAPTER 15

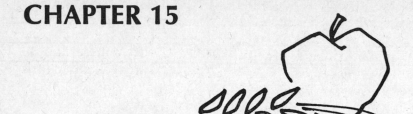

NEW WAYS TO EAT AWAY GOUT AND ARTHRITIS

So far in this book, we've been talking about WHAT we eat—food and nutrition. But HOW we eat—the very act of eating itself—also plays a major role in recovery from arthritis and gout. Some cases of arthritic disease may actually be caused more by *how* we eat than by *what* we eat.

For example, we can greatly reduce exposure to Allergy Foods by rotating our diet and by eating mini-meals instead of the usual three "squares" a day. And we can often improve our digestion (and reduce risk of arthritis) by using food to restore the acid-alkiline balance of our body chemistry.

By improving the way we eat, as well as what we eat, our arthritis therapy becomes more Holistic.

How to Eat Allergy Foods Safely Again

You may not have to stop eating all Allergy Foods permanently. By adding more variety to your diet, so that servings of Allergy Foods are spaced farther apart, you can very probably start to eat most of these foods again after a few weeks of abstinence.

The fact is that most of us simply don't eat the variety of foods that we should. Experiments have proved that when the body is in optimum health balance and free of all nutritional stress, we will naturally choose foods containing the nutrients we need.

But once the body's self-regulatory mechanisms are distorted by Stressor Foods, we choose foods like sugar and fats that contribute to allergies.

Instead of eating a wide assortment of foods, we avoid diversification and keep on eating the same foods over and over. Most people eat only 12–16 different foods. As we continually eat large and frequent amounts of just a few foods, we become addicted to these foods and constantly crave them.

Ease of preparation also guides people to eat, say, bread which is immediately available instead of waiting 30 minutes to bake some vegetables. If physical activity is restricted by arthritis, our choice of foods may be narrowed even more by inability to move around and shop.

Thus we continue to eat a relatively few foods, and we often eat a single food several times a day. Our modern trucking industry allows us to keep these same foods on the table every day of the year.

But in Nature, foods change with the season. Primitive man found a variety of alternative and different foods that provided a perfect nutritional balance.

By adding more variety to your diet and eating more kinds of different foods, you may very well be able to once again begin eating certain foods to which you have an allergy. This is possible because there are two types of food allergies.

- *Fixed Allergies* are innate and may be caused by a genetic intolerance. They will always be with us. No matter how long you abstain from a food or how little you may eat, an allergic reaction will always occur.

- *Cyclical Allergies* are an acquired rejection response that develops as the results of nutritional or other stress.

Fortunately, Cyclical Allergies are by far the more common. The only way to ascertain which type you have is to abstain from an allergenic food for several weeks, then to eat a fairly large amount at a single meal. If no reaction occurs, it is probably a Cyclical Allergy.

The Astounding Rotation System for Overcoming Allergies

After an abstinence of six weeks or more, Cyclical Allergy Foods can be re-introduced into the diet provided that:

- You eat no Allergy Food more often than once every 5 days.
- You eat no Allergy Food from any one family more often than every other day.
- Not more than one Allergy Food should be eaten on any one day.

Let's say you have Cyclical Allergies to wheat, corn, veal, chicken and peanuts. After abstaining from these foods for six weeks, you become temporarily desensitized to them.

Within the guidelines just described, you may then try re-introducing each of these foods back into your diet. For example, you could eat wheat on Monday, veal on Tuesday, corn on Wednesday, chicken on Thursday and peanuts on Friday. In this way, the two grass family cereals are spaced two days apart. (Food families are listed in Chapter 7.)

The rest of your food doesn't have to be on a 5-day rotational basis. You can eat non-allergenic foods more often. But to discourage any possible tendency to future allergies, it is wise to rotate your foods and to eat as many widely different foods as you can.

Some people may have multiple allergies to as many as ten or even 15 different foods. If you have this many Cyclical Allergies, you must still space them out so that only one Allergy Food is eaten each day. Should you try to eat normal-sized helpings of two or more allergenic foods in one day, the total allergenic exposure could well be sufficient to trigger the immune response and cause an arthritis flare-up.

If you desire to eat two allergenic foods in one day, then eat only half a serving of each.

A Sample Five Day Rotation Menu

Here is a sample menu in which the five Allergy Foods (in capitals) are rotated on a 5-day basis.

Day	Breakfast	Lunch	Dinner
1	Canteloupe	Vegetable salad	Vegetable salad
	Honeydew	Yogurt	Baked haddock
	Watermelon	WHOLE	Potatoes, parsnips,
		WHEAT	peas, onions
		BREAD	

Day	Breakfast	Lunch	Dinner
2	Apple	Vegetable salad	Vegetable salad
	Pear	VEAL	Baked cod
	Apricot	Baked potatoes	Brown rice
	Peach	Green beans	Steamed vegetables
			Navy beans
3	Grapes	Vegetable salad	Vegetable salad
	Apricots	Soybeans	Baked haddock
	Apples	PEANUTS	Rutabagas
		Sunflower and	Turnips
		sesame seeds	Beans
		Mixed nuts	Peas
			Onions
4	Bananas	Vegetable salad	Vegetable salad
	Apricots	Baked haddock	Brown rice
	Peaches	CORN	wok-prepared
		Green beans	vegetables
5	Pineapple	Vegetable salad	Vegetable salad
	Cooked oatmeal	CHICKEN	Vegetable soup
		Baked potato	Sweet potatoes
		Peas	White beans
			Onions

Although the menu contains more cooked vegetables than is perhaps ideal, it still meets the 80-10-10 guidelines because of the large vegetable salads that precede each lunch and dinner. Salad vegetables would be varied as much as possible to include sprouts, tomatoes and avocados.

As Restorative Foods rebuild total health, sensitivities to Cyclical Allergy Foods may gradually disappear altogether. But this can take a year or more. Meanwhile, use a Rotational Menu to space out Cyclical Allergy Foods so that you can continue to eat them without triggering a rejectivity response.

The Reverend C. Eats Allergy Foods Safely Once More

The Reverend C. had suffered from rheumatoid arthritis since his early fifties. When he retired at 65, he took time off to enroll at a Holistically oriented arthritic clinic. There he fasted for

5 days and tested allergy-positive to sugar, corn, oats, beef, milk and cheese.

Recovery was gradual but steady. Three months later, Reverend C. was able to walk for several miles and to swim and ride a bicycle.

After phoning the arthritis clinic, Reverend C. was advised to try re-introducing corn and oats back into his diet. Since both were grass family cereals, he was advised to eat each once every 4 days and to eat them only on alternate days. This meant that during a 4-day cycle, Reverend C. ate corn the first day and oats on the third day.

By carefully observing this rotational technique, Reverend C. found that he could eat two ears of corn on the first day and a large bowl of oatmeal on the third day without any hint of arthritis symptoms.

Poor Digestion May Be Causing Arthritis

Poor digestion is the most common symptom of a food allergy. Almost everyone with a severe food allergy suffers from some degree of gastro-intestinal trouble whenever they eat the allergenic food.

Strangely, however, instead of the allergy causing poor digestion, it may be the other way around.

Faulty chewing and improper eating can lead to incomplete digestion. When food is not fully digested, the number of undigested food particles increases. When these many more particles are absorbed into the bloodstream, they rapidly set off an immune response and trigger arthritis. Thus the poorer the digestion, the greater the risk of rheumatoid and similar forms of arthritis.

Most nutritionists believe that poor chewing and improper eating habits can actually cause rheumatoid arthritis. In any event, you can benefit both your arthritis and your digestion by learning the rules of successful eating.

Improper mastication and faulty digestion are the usual causes of bloating, excess gas, heartburn, indigestion, acid stomach and many cases of constipation and diarrhea. When enzymes are lacking, as in cooked foods, food is often poorly absorbed and much of its nutrient value is lost.

By obeying the rules of successful digestion below, you can

speed your recovery from arthritis or gout by 20 per cent and often more.

What we've been talking about so far in this book concerns food and nutrition. The rules below govern the act of eating.

Rules for Eating Away Gout and Arthritis

Never Overeat or Stuff Yourself.
Avoid Large Meals. Eat Mini-Meals Instead.

The smaller your meals, the less the body is stressed and the more stable are your self-regulatory systems. This reduces your risk of food allergies and arthritic disease. It doesn't seem to matter how frequent your meals are, provided they are smaller.

A two year study of 4,057 people aged 20 and over by Dr. Allen B. Nichols at the University of Michigan revealed that eating larger meals can be as dangerous to the heart and blood vessels as a high-fat diet. Whenever a large meal is eaten, the body is stressed with a sudden surge of sugar and fat. People who eat large meals must process and store twice as much fat and sugar as those who eat sparingly. These heavy eaters build up stomachs and intestines that are 40 per cent larger than in normal eaters.

Eating 3 large "square" meals daily also increases the quantity and capacity of fat cells and leads to rapid weight gain.

Although arthritis and gout have not been directly linked to heavy eating, other degenerative diseases have. Eating large meals has been proved to lead to heart disease, maturity diabetes and hypertension and, by suppressing the immune system, to cancer. Since all degenerative diseases have the same cause, it appears extremely likely that heavy eating is also a causative factor in the onset of arthritis and gout.

For example, at Prague University, Czechoslovakia, Dr. Paul Fabry conducted a study of 1,133 men aged 60–64. He found that heart disease was significantly greater among those who ate 3 or fewer meals a day (30.5 per cent had heart attacks) than among those who consumed the same amount spread over 5 meals or more (only 20 per cent had heart attacks).

Research has shown that primitive human populations seldom if ever ate large, heavy meals. Instead, they nibbled small amounts of food at frequent intervals.

Our bodies are simply not adapted to handling the stress of coping with large, heavy meals. When Dr. Grant Gwineup, a professor at the University of California at Irvine, changed meal patterns from 3 standard-sized meals a day to 10 Mini-Meals, he found that the reduced stress significantly reduced risk of heart attack.

The Wizardry of Mini-Meals

Many cardiac rehabilitation centers break each standard-sized meal into 3 Mini-Meals and serve a total of 9 small meals spread over the day. Records kept at these institutions show that obese people who change to eating Mini-Meals lose approximately two pounds per week without reducing their calorie intake. In less than 3 months, their serum cholesterol level has frequently returned to normal. The records also show that while recovering from heart disease through Mini-Meals, some patients have simultaneously recovered from both osteo- and rheumatoid arthritis and from gout.

To eat the Mini-Meal way, you take your usual breakfast and divide it into 3 equal portions. You do the same with your usual lunch and dinner. This provides 9 Mini-Meals which you eat throughout the day at approximately 90 minute intervals.

If you prefer, you can divide your normal daily ration into as few as 5 Mini-Meals. Or into any larger number you wish. Of course, you still observe the other rules such as eating only when calm and when hungry, and you must still eat slowly and chew each mouthful thoroughly.

People who work find few problems in dovetailing Mini-Meals into most job schedules. You can begin with one Mini-Meals at breakfast time, a second during the mid-morning break, a third at lunchtime, a fourth during the mid-afternoon break, a fifth immediately upon reaching home and the rest spread over the evening. You can easily carry fresh, raw foods to work such as nuts, seeds, fruits, salad vegetables and whole grain bread.

Eating the Mini-Meal way virtually guarantees freedom from bloating, gas or indigestion. The meals are so light that digestion is scarcely noticeable and you are permanently freed from ever feeling logy or distressingly full. Observations have shown that absorption is far better, and the pulse rate seldom rises when small meals are eaten.

There is also a growing body of evidence to show that allergenic foods eaten the Mini-Meal way are less likely to set off the immune response and to bring on arthritis.

No one with gout or arthritis should fail to change over to the Mini-Meal way of eating.

Eat Only When Hungry

Much of our eating is done for entertainment or amusement or as a social habit or to relieve boredom or as a stimulant. From now on, eat only when you are actually hungry. If you are not actually hungry, skip a meal.

Eat Only When You Feel Calm and Serene and When the Atmosphere Is Peaceful and Relaxed

Never eat when you are tired, tense, sick, upset or late at night.

If you feel hungry or emotionally tense at the same time, use this quick-relaxation technique. Stand upright and tense all the muscles in the body simultaneously. Hold for 8 seconds. Then release. Tense your arms, legs, hands, feet, abdomen, back, neck and face muscles. If you can't tense them all at once, tense both arms and hands first, hold to the slow count of 8, and release. Then repeat with both legs, with the shoulders and back, with the abdomen and buttocks, and with the neck and face.

Next sit or lie down and take six slow, deep breaths. Inhale for 4 seconds, hold the breath for 4 seconds, and exhale for 4 seconds. Take six of these slow, deep inhalations. Then relax and visualize yourself running along a beach with your spine and joints as flexible as a kitten's and with all your arthritis already gone. Keep visualizing yourself as already recovered from arthritis.

By the time your mind tires of this exercise, you will be completely calm and serene and ready to eat.

Eat Slowly and Chew Foods Well

Never eat on the run or against the clock or when in a hurry or while standing up. These are almost certain ways to develop an allergy. A good way to slow down your eating is to use chopsticks.

Digestion of all starches and other complex carbohydrates

begins in the mouth. The food must be thoroughly chewed and mixed with saliva. Swallow each mouthful only when it is chewed into a liquid pulp.

Failing to thoroughly chew beans is the reason why many people complain that these foods cause flatulence. (If you still find that beans are gassy, try cooking them together with brown rice.)

You will also lose weight faster by eating slowly and chewing more. This is because after eating it takes about ten minutes for a feeling of fullness to register in the brain. By eating more slowly you will feel full before you have eaten as much food.

Avoid Drinking Liquids with Meals

Drinking liquids with meals dilutes stomach acids and digestive enzymes and inhibits the entire digestive process. You can avoid this problem by not drinking within 20 minutes of eating a standard-sized meal nor for 90 minutes afterwards. With Mini-Meals, avoid drinking for ten minutes before eating and for 30 minutes after finishing.

Eat Sparingly but Enjoy It

Several studies on longevity have all found that people who eat sparingly live longer and enjoy better health. As we have already learned, people with optimum health do not get arthritis or gout.

Here are several simple techniques that will almost ensure you eat sparingly.

- Before beginning any meal, throw away one fifth of the food on your plate. Then try to leave some food on your plate when you finish.

- After a meal is served, sit and wait a full minute before starting to eat.

- Put down the utensils between each mouthful until it is completely chewed and swallowed. Or if eating with your hands, put your food back on the plate after each bite.

- Bite off or take only a half a mouthful at a time instead of a full mouthful.

- If you are right-handed, eat with the left hand. Or vice versa. This will slow down your eating.
- Keep the refrigerator almost empty.
- Always leave the table feeling slightly hungry.

June R. Loses Her Arthritis by Eating Holistically

When June R. used several eating techniques simultaneously in a Holistic approach to healing arthritis, she achieved dynamic results.

"I had osteo-arthritis and my problem was fifty pounds of surplus fat," June told me on the patio of her Arizona retirement home. "This was when I worked in an ad agency and my busy schedule left no time for fasting. I had never been able to stick with any diet. Finally, I signed up with a weight-loss clinic that specialized in behavior motivation.

"I was instructed to eat a low-fat, high-fiber diet of fresh, natural foods and I had to prepare it in the eighty-ten-ten way. Well, I was allowed to eat as much as I wanted provided I ate it in the form of nine small meals each spaced ninety minutes apart. I could eat only when I felt hungry and I was to chew each mouthful thoroughly before swallowing. I also agreed to eat only when I felt emotionally calm and relaxed."

All of June's previous diets had stressed low carbohydrate consumption and had left her feeling hungry and tired. This time it was different. She found her complex carbohydrate diet so filling that she actually had to skip two Mini-Meals each day.

"I never felt hungry and I ate all I wanted," June said. "But I still lost a steady five pounds a week. This Holistic approach was a powerful system. Without ever counting calories or feeling hungry, in three months my weight dropped right back to normal.

"With every pound I lost, my knees felt better. By the time I was back in a size twelve dress, I was able to walk without any pain and I could even dance.

"I've stayed faithfully with the natural foods diet and the Mini-Meals, and I've never changed the eighty-ten-ten formula. All that super-nutrition gradually restored health to my knees.

Right now at sixty-five, I'm as flexible and agile as when I was twenty-one. My weight is exactly what it was then. And I don't have a trace of arthritis.''

How to Tell If Your Body Chemistry Is in Balance

A frequent cause of poor digestion in people with arthritic disease is an insufficiency of hydrochloric acid in the stomach. The acid helps break down and digest food. When there isn't sufficient acid, gas and other forms of intestinal blitz may occur. But lack of stomach acid can increase the number of undigested food particles and increase risk of arthritis.

This condition often shows up as an alkalinity in the urine. You can check the pH or acid-alkaline balance of your urine by purchasing a small roll of Phenaphthazine paper sold in health food stores. Clip a half inch strip of the paper in a clothes pin and dip into a specimen of your urine. It will immediately change color. By comparing it with a color chart that comes with the paper, you can read off the pH of your urine.

The paper registers pH from 4.5 to 7.5. Anything above 7 is alkaline. Below 7, the paper shows varying degrees of acidity. During daytime, the urine is usually acidic with a normal reading of about 5.8. While sleeping, alkalinity increases as the body detoxifies itself. A peak of toxemia occurs around 4 a.m., after which the acid tide returns.

Test your urine immediately upon rising and again about an hour after breakfast. The first reading will show if the acid tide has been restored after the nightly detoxification. The second should show a gradually increasing acidity. Take another reading in mid-afternoon as a check.

An alkaline pH during the daytime may be associated with a chronic disease or with being weak or run down. People with gout or arthritis often have an alkaline daytime pH.

An insufficiency of stomach acid often leads to body-wide alkalinity because acid foods are changed during ingestion into alkaline end products.

If the urine tests alkaline during the daytime, it is telling us that we have an insufficiency of stomach acid or that we are eating too many acid fruits or both. This is because acid fruits are changed during digestion into alkaline end products. They then add to the body's overall alkalinity that is usually caused in the first place by a deficiency of hydrochloric acid in the stomach.

Acid foods include such fruits as citrus, pineapple, tomato, sour plum and strawberries. Somewhat less acidic are apples, apricots, cherries, grapes, blueberries, peaches, plums, raspberries, and several tropical fruits like chirimoya, mango and papaya.

By comparison, the most alkaline foods are grains. Upon digestion, their end products are alkaline.

Grains can, therefore, be used to neutralize the effect of acid fruits. By eating somewhat fewer acid fruits and by replacing them with grains, we can usually swing any daytime alkaline balance in the urine over to the acid side.

In any event, avoid eating too much fruit. As recommended earlier, always try to eat at least twice as much vegetables as fruit.

A common symptom associated with over-alkalinity is frequent nocturnal urination. (If you have not already done so, check with your doctor to make sure this is not due to an infection or to an enlarged prostate in males.) If you wake up often during the night to void, and are unable to get back to sleep for 30 minutes or more, this may be a food allergy symptom.

Using Food to Rebalance
Your Body Chemistry

You can compensate for over-alkalinity by eating fewer acidic fruits and by eating more grains. Usually only minor changes are necessary—perhaps eating one or two fewer acid fruits and adding one or two extra slices of whole grain bread. Don't try to keep your pH below 5. A reading of 5.8 is ideal.

Naturally, your pH will vary depending on the food and drink you have recently consumed. What you're aiming for is an overall long-term average of 5.8. You can't expect to keep it at 5.8 all of the time. If your urine is steadily alkaline during the daytime, it may be due to a still-undetected food allergy.

By restoring the normal pH of your urine, you are improving your digestion and thereby reducing the risk of auto-immune attack on arthritic joints.

Sane Eating Helps Donna C.
Lose Her Arthritis

Donna C. had suffered with rheumatoid arthritis in her hands, knees and ankles for over 5 years. Her arthritis seemed to be linked to poor digestion. Whenever she had an upset stomach, the following day her arthritis would flare up.

One summer, Donna decided to spend 3 weeks at a health resort attending a seminar on eating and nutrition. Among the many things she learned were the rules for proper eating. Donna was also taught to balance her body chemistry by using food to normalize the pH of her urine.

Donna found that her urine was strongly alkaline at all times. Each night she had to get up at least once and go to the bathroom.

Donna discovered she was addicted to eating a grapefruit at the start of each meal. She dropped two of these daily citrus fruits and added two thick slices of whole wheat bread instead. She also divided up her three standard daily meals into nine Mini-Meals and she omitted all Stressor Foods from her diet.

It took only 4 days for Donna's pH to become acidic and to drop to a more normal reading of 5.8. As it did so, she began to feel better. The arthritis pain gradually subsided and she found she had to get up less often at night.

After a week on Mini-Meals, Donna's digestive problems also disappeared. As long as she stayed with the Mini-Meals and kept her pH normal, Donna had no further trouble with either arthritis or indigestion.

When she phoned the nutritionist at the health resort to describe her success, he said that Donna had probably been allergic to citrus and to some of the Stressor Foods she had cut out of her diet. When the cause of her arthritis and digestive problems was removed, her body quickly healed itself.

As Donna C. discovered, we have a fountain of health and youth already within us. Through harmful habits of eating and living, we turn the fountain off. Yet we can always turn the fountain on again by replacing our health-destroying eating and living habits and with beneficial health-restoring foods . . . and by cultivating other habits designed to produce high-level wellness.

That is the message of the Holistic approach to healing described in this book. Through learning all about gout and arthritis and about *all* the options and alternatives available—not merely medical options—we can each become a medically-educated layperson thoroughly capable of taking control of our own health and taking an active role in our own recovery.

No drug, injection or treatment can tap our wellsprings of inner health. Only we ourselves can turn on the recuperative and rejuvenative powers that lie within us. In the final analysis, overcoming gout or arthritis is something that only we can do for ourselves.

DICTIONARY OF RESTORATIVE FOODS

Although arthritis and gout are caused by eating harmful Stressor Foods, and both diseases can be reversed by changing to a diet of natural, Restorative Foods, this does not mean that natural foods are medicines.

A basic law of holistic healing is that only the body can heal. Neither drugs nor foods can heal. Healing is a biological process that can be accomplished only by the body's own recuperative and rejuvenative powers. Drugs can be helpful in emergency situations such as when the immune system is overwhelmed by rapidly-multiplying armies of invading bacteria. Antibiotics will destroy the bacteria hordes, allowing the body's white cells to regain control. But any damage done by the bacteria is healed by the body's own cells, not by the drug.

When the cause of disease is removed, the body becomes a self-healing entity provided it is supplied with its biological necessities. These include pure air and water, rest, emotional calm and natural, nutrient-rich foods.

The Restorative Foods described below are foods the body needs to supply the energy, minerals, vitamins, chlorophyll, enzymes and protein required in the healing process. These Restorative Foods are essential to the healing process. But it is the body that is doing the healing, not the foods.

This perspective is important in understanding the role of food in healing and in avoiding the common mistake of regarding specific foods as medicines.

To ensure that the body assimilates and utilizes these Restorative Foods—thereby maximizing the healing process—they should ideally be eaten in proper combinations. The basic rules for proper food combining are outlined in Chapter 11. If, however, you experience any gas, flatulence or other form of indigestion after eating combinations of vegetables or of fruits, you can probably avoid it in future by observing the following, more detailed rules for successful food combining.

Protein foods combine well with green vegetables and with acid fruits but not with starches or sweet fruits.

Starchy vegetables combine well with other starches, including most cereals.

Green vegetables combine well with vegetables, proteins and starches but not with most fruits.

Cereals, mostly grains, combine well with most green and starchy vegetables and with fats. They are not always compatible with fruits, especially acid fruits. However, most sub-acid and sweet fruits may be safely mixed with most breakfast cereals.

Acid fruits combine reasonably well with sub-acid fruits and with protein but should not be mixed with starches.

Sub-acid fruits combine reasonably well with acid fruits and may be mixed in reasonable amounts with breakfast cereals or dairy foods.

Sweet fruits combine well with sub-acid fruits but not with acid fruits. They do not mix well with proteins.

Neutral fruits mix well with sub-acid fruits and with green vegetables.

All the Restorative Foods in the following list are identified by food class so that you may combine them properly. All foods of the same type are compatible and may be safely mixed and eaten together. (*Example:* broccoli, Brussels sprouts, cabbage, cauliflower, celery, chard, chives, collards and cucumber are all classified as green vegetables and can be safely eaten together at the same meal.)

Most natural foods also belong to food families based on their origin. For example, most melons, pumpkins, cucumbers and squash are descendents of the gourd and belong to the gourd family. Since all foods belonging to any one family are genetically similar, when a person develops an allergy to one food they often are allergic to other foods of the same family.

The significance of food families in tracking down allergies is described in Chapter 7. To assist you in identifying other members of any food family to which you may be allergic, the family to which each food belongs is (where known) listed below.

While all foods which follow are nutritionally helpful to the body in recovering from arthritic disease, you should not eat any to which you know you are allergic.

Acerola (Barbados Cherry). This red-fluted cherry grows on hedges and bushes in South Florida. It is delicious when eaten raw. Since the acerola is a phenomenally rich source of Vitamin C, it is of great value in helping the body overcome the aching and swelling of arthritic joints. (A close relative is the pitanga or Surinam cherry.) Class: *acid fruit*.

Almond: plum family. Fresh, whole, shelled almonds are rich in protein and are a good source of potassium, magnesium, calcium and phosphorus. Almonds go well with vegetable salads or with citrus. Class: *protein*.

Apple: apple family. Eaten unpeeled, apples aid the body in healing arthritis by supplying essential pepsin. When fresh apples are unavailable, dried apples may be eaten; they are also a good substitute for candy. Apple cider vinegar appears to benefit the digestive system and fresh apple juice makes a pleasant drink. However, most nutrients in apple butter and apple jelly have been lost through processing. Class: *sub-acid fruit*.

Apricot: plum family. This delicious fruit is rich in iron and other minerals. Dried apricots are acceptable if free of preservatives like sulphur dioxide. To avoid cooking, soften them in water overnight. Class: *sub-acid fruit* (sweet fruit when dried).

Artichoke: aster family. The several varieties of this tuber, including the French and Jerusalem artichoke, are good sources of potassium, iron, magnesium and calcium as well as Vitamins A and C and the B-complex. They can be eaten raw or briefly baked or steamed. Class: *starchy vegetable*.

Asparagus: lily family. These succulent shoots supply nutrients which the body uses in purifying muscle cells and kidneys, an essential step in overall recovery from arthritis. Asparagus shoots may be eaten raw or lightly steamed for a few minutes, after which they should be eaten promptly before they become limp and lose taste. Class: *green vegetable*.

Avocado: laurel family. This versatile food, available in different varieties through much of the year, combines well with both fruits and vegetables. It is ripe when slightly soft and may be mixed into fruit or vegetable salads or used as a spread on celery sticks or on whole grain bread. The avocado supplies cholesterol-free fat and is rich in essential nutrients needed by the body during recovery from arthritis. Class: *neutral fruit*.

Bamboo shoots: grass family. Bamboo shoot tips are frequently obtainable in oriental food shops. They are valued by Chinese and Japanese as an aid to the body in expelling toxins and in helping lower blood pressure. They may be eaten raw or cooked for a few minutes. Class: *starchy vegetable*.

Banana: banana family. Bananas are one of the best sources of potassium, a nutrient essential to the body during the healing process. Bananas speckled with brown dots are the most ripe and sweet; partly green ones are often starchy and may not ripen fully. Besides being used in fruit salads or eaten on bread, bananas may be frozen to form a natural ice cream. A larger variety with angular sides, the plantain, is often baked. Class: *sweet fruit*.

Barley: grass family. Only unpearled (unrefined) barley should be eaten. It can be cooked as a breakfast cereal (one cup of barley to 4 cups of water) with raisins added while cooking. Barley is a good source of energy and B vitamins. Class: *cereal*.

Beans: legume family. The best way to eat beans is to sprout them. Otherwise, they should be cooked by gentle simmering in a bean crock. Approximately 20 per cent of the content of dried beans is protein. Soybeans are an important source of iron, potassium and unsaturated fatty acids, while butter and lima beans also abound with vitamins and minerals, especially iron. Mung beans, used exclusively for sprouting, supply a wide assortment of vitamins and minerals which are often deficient in persons suffering from arthritis. String beans are also rich in calcium, magnesium and potassium. **Alfalfa,** an important food in arthritis recovery, is also a legume. Class: *protein*.

Beechnut: beech family. This small northern nut is high in vegetable protein, unsaturated fatty acids and energy. Class: *protein*.

Beet: goosefoot family. Beets are best eaten raw after being grated and sprinkled on vegetable salads. They may also be lightly steamed or baked. The nutritional value of cooked beets may be enhanced by lightly steaming the beet greens, which are rich in iron and other vital minerals, and eating them with the beets. Either raw, or cooked with the greens, beets supply important nutrients used by the body in recovery from arthritis and especially from gout. Class: *starchy vegetable*.

Blackberry: rose family. Nutrients in this berry, which grows on wild brambles in cool, northern areas, are utilized by the body in purifying the bloodstream and digestive tract during recovery from arthritic disease. Blueberries and loganberries have similar nutritional qualities. The berries should be eaten raw; they are delicious with breakfast cereals. Class: *sub-acid fruits*.

Brazil nut: sapucaia family. This South American import is high in calcium, phosphorus, iron, vegetable protein, calories and unsaturated fat. Class: *protein*.

Broccoli: cruciferous family. When the small green heads are chopped up in a salad they supply nutrients which aid the body in rebalancing its carbohydrate metabolism. Alternatively, broccoli may be split and lightly steamed. Class: *green vegetable*.

Brussels sprouts: cruciferous family. Sprouts taste best when about an inch in diameter. Chop and mix them in a raw vegetable salad; or steam for 8–10 minutes. They supply nutrients which aid the body in rebalancing its carbohydrate metabolism. Class: *green vegetable*.

Buckwheat: buckwheat family. Because real buckwheat is often highly refined in milling, most "buckwheat" is actually a mix of corn, rye, wheat and other grains. It is nonetheless quite desirable. Class: *cereal*.

Buttermilk: bovid family. This low-fat dairy food is a fine source of protein, calcium, potassium, phosphorus and riboflavin, a B vitamin. Class: *protein*.

Cabbage: cruciferous family. The numerous varieties of early and late, green and purple cabbage are good sources of iron, calcium and other nutrients used by the body in expelling toxins during recovery from gout or arthritis. Cabbage is delicious when raw, especially the purple type. The outer leaves are richest in calcium, so don't discard them. Cabbage may also be cooked lightly till crisp but never, as many restaurants do, till soggy. Class: *green vegetable*.

Cactus fruit: tuna family. Widely available in the Southwest and Mexico, where it is called the tuna or prickly pear, cactus fruit is a tasty, natural food. It must be peeled before eating. Class: *sub-acid fruit*.

Canistel (eggfruit). This soft, yellow tropical fruit is fairly common in South Florida and is a valuable source of Vitamin C. Class: *sweet fruit*.

Carambola. This oval, five-sided tropical fruit is often seen in South Florida. It is rich in vitamins and minerals utilized by the body in purifying and healing. Class: *acid fruit.*

Carob: legume family. The pods of the carob tree may be eaten as fruit. More commonly, they are ground into carob powder and sold in health food stores for making a healthful beverage or as a chocolate substitute. Carob powder is a good source of Vitamin A and the B-complex plus calcium, iron, copper, and magnesium. Be sure any carob you buy is sugar-free. Class: *sweet fruit.*

Carrot: parsley family. Eaten raw, carrots supply the body with Vitamin A and other nutrients which are utilized in restoring balance to the immune system and endocrine glands. Small, young carrots are best for eating raw; they may be eaten whole or grated, sliced or shredded. Larger, older carrots may be steamed, mashed or made into a soup. Class: *starchy vegetable.*

Cashew nut: cashew family. This desirable nut is sold shelled because an acid in the shell can blister flesh. In shelling, the nuts are twice heated to 350°F hence they are more liable to rancidity than most other nuts. Class: *protein.*

Cauliflower: cruciferous family. Best chopped up fine while raw and added to a vegetable salad, cauliflower contains nutrients utilized by the body in restoring carbohydrate metabolism. Older people, who may find difficulty digesting the cauliflower raw, may steam it briefly. Class: *green vegetable.*

Celery: parsley family. Eaten whole along with the leaves or chopped in a salad, raw celery is a good source of calcium and other important nutrients utilized by the body during recovery from arthritis and other degenerative diseases. Class: *green vegetable.*

Chard: goosefoot family. Chard leaves are high in potassium, calcium, iron and Vitamin A and when eaten raw supply the body with nutrients utilized during arthritis recovery. Class: *green vegetable.*

Cherry: plum family. Raw cherries supply iron, magnesium and other nutrients required by the body while restoring health following arthritis and gout or other degenerative diseases. The darker the cherries, the richer they are in iron and magnesium. Cherries in pies and preserves have lost much of their nutritional value. Class: *sub-acid fruit.*

Chestnut: beech family. A good source of iron and phosphorus, chestnuts are difficult to digest raw owing to their tannic acid content. Lightly roasted, they make a delicious addition to vegetable salads or to chicken or turkey served with sweet potatoes. Class: *protein*.

Chicken: quail family. Chicken eaten without the skin is a desirable low fat source of whole protein and is also high in phosphorus and potassium. Class: *protein*.

Chives: lily family. The slender leaves of this onion plant are chopped fine and used to flavor salads and soups. Class: *green vegetable*.

Citrus: citrus family. All members of the citrus family—oranges, grapefruit, lemons, limes, tangerines and tangelos—are good sources of Vitamin C while the pith contains bio-flavinoids which help in keeping the arteries flexible. Citrus supplies the body with nutrients utilized in breaking up calcium deposits in arthritic joints. Drinking fresh juice is slightly less desirable than eating the fruit. However, the juice of limes or lemons makes a tasty addition to herb teas, to vegetable and fruit salads and to tropical fruits. Class: *acid fruit*.

Coconut: palm family. This large nut is a good source of fat and protein but both the coconut and all coconut products contain cholesterol. Coconut, if eaten, should be whole and fresh. Drain out the water and drink it. Green coconuts sold in Florida have meat that is so soft, it can be eaten with a spoon. Older, harder coconut meat can be cut up and eaten like other nuts or grated and sprinkled on vegetable salads. Class: *protein*.

Cod: cod family. A superior source of low-fat protein, this valuable food fish also supplies phosphorus and potassium. Highly recommended. Class: *protein*.

Collards: cruciferous family. This headless cabbage is an important source of calcium and other nutrients required by the body in healing gout or arthritis. The leaves can be eaten raw in a salad or lightly steamed for a few minutes. Class: *green vegetable*.

Corn: grass family. Eaten raw when young or briefly steamed when mature, corn is a valuable body-building staple. The fact that it is classified as a vegetable when young and fresh, and as a starchy cereal when older and dried indicates that young, fresh corn eaten raw is less likely to be allergenic. Unfortunately, corn products such as corn syrup, meal or starch are denatured by heat during manufacture while hominy, another form of corn, may be contaminated by chemicals used in removing its outer shell. Class: *vegetable* when fresh and young; *cereal* when older and dried.

Cottage cheese: bovid family. Low-fat cottage cheese is a superior source of whole protein and a good source of calcium, Vitamins B_6 and B_{12}, phosphorus, and riboflavin. It makes a splendid salad dressing and also blends well with sub-acid fruits. Class: *protein*.

Cranberry: heath family. Too tart and acidic to eat raw, the cranberry must be lightly cooked. Because large amounts of sugar are added to commercially prepared cranberries, home preparation is recommended. Even cooked, the cranberry is a valuable source of essential nutrients used by the body in recovering from gout. Class: *acid fruit*.

Cucumber: gourd family. High in potassium and other minerals, this watery vegetable is a mild diuretic. A mixture of fresh cucumber and carrot juice aids the body in purifying itself of uric acid. Pickled cucumbers are nutritionally valueless. Try, also, to buy cucumbers that have not had their skins oiled by supermarket employees. Class: *green vegetable*.

Currant: gooseberry family. Of the three varieties of currant—red, black and white—the red is richest in minerals. Currants mixed with freshly grated coconut and rolled into balls make a fine natural candy. Class: *acid fruit*.

Dandelion greens: aster family. The small, young leaves of cultivated varieties like the Improved Broad Leaf are a welcome addition to salads. Wild dandelions are rather too bitter. Dandelions can also be cooked like spinach. Raw dandelions, or dandelion tea, contain nutrients valuable to the body in restoring health. Class: *green vegetable*.

Date: palm family. Good sources of iron and potassium, dates are an excellent substitute for candy. They should be eaten in limited amounts because they are rapidly absorbed and flood the bloodstream with sugar. Class: *sweet fruit*.

Dulse: This American salt water algae is an important source of iron, calcium, iodine and phosphorus. The dried, purple leaves are sold in most health food stores and they impart a zesty tang when chopped and sprinkled on salads or other foods. The leaves may also be chewed alone and are nutritionally superior to the powdered or tablet form of dulse.

Eggplant: nightshade family. Baked together with tomatoes and garlic, this purple vegetable provides a tasty dish. It contains nutrients used by the body in restoring sound digestion. Class: *green vegetable*.

Endives: aster family. The broad leafed variety of endive is also known as escarole. Endive should be chopped and mixed into a green salad since it is rather bitter when eaten alone. A good source of potassium, calcium and phosphorus, it supplies essential nutrients utilized by the body in rebalancing carbohydrate metabolism. Class: *green vegetable*.

Fig: mulberry family. Their high iron and mineral content makes figs nutritionally valuable to the body in its efforts to cleanse the bowels and restore sound digestion. Fresh figs are preferable. Dried figs make a good substitute for candy but should be eaten only in limited quantities due to their rapid absorption and release of sugar into the bloodstream. Class: *sweet fruit*.

Filbert: beech family. Known also as the hazelnut or cobnut, the filbert has a high content of calcium and phosphorus and is a good source of cholesterol-free fat and protein. Class: *protein*.

Garlic: lily family. The cloves of this hardy bulb supply essential nutrients used by the body in self-purification and in restoring balance to the lymph and digestive systems. Add chopped cloves to stews and steamed dishes or rub them over a wooden salad bowl before filling. Health food stores also sell squeezers for extracting the juice from garlic cloves. It can be dripped into almost any kind of cooked food. Garlic oil is also available in capsules. Powdered garlic is considered nutritionally inferior. Class: *vegetable*.

Gooseberry: gooseberry family. Eaten raw, this delicious northern berry supplies nutrients valuable to the body in restoring balance to several functions of body chemistry involved in arthritis recovery. Class: *acid fruit*.

Grape: grape family. Valued for nutrients used by the body in excreting uric acid, raw, fresh grapes are delicious when eaten alone or in a fruit salad. Raisins, which are dried grapes, and which have a high mineral content, are equally desirable and may be added to many foods to impart added flavor. Fresh grape juice is a commendable beverage. Class: *sub-acid fruit*.

Guava: myrtle family. The apple of the tropics, the guava grows wild in South Florida. Although the guava is used in jams, jellies and paste, it is best when eaten raw; simply peel it and munch. The guava contains nutrients utilized by the body in restoring health to the circulatory system. Class: *sub-acid fruit*.

Haddock: cod family. A fillet of this deep ocean fish supplies 18.3 grams of whole protein yet only .1 grams of fat. The haddock is also a dependable source of calcium, potassium, phosphorus and magnesium. Class: *protein*.

Kale: cruciferous family. The curled, wrinkled leaves of this headless cabbage are rich in nutrients utilized by the body during recovery from arthritic disease. Kale is best eaten raw in salads, or it may be lightly steamed. Class: *green vegetable*.

Kelp: This seaweed is an important source of iron, calcium, phosphorus and iodine as well as vegetable protein. It is usually eaten as a zesty seasoning sprinkled on salads and other foods.

Kohlrabi: cruciferous family. When peeled, this white, nutty vegetable may be eaten raw or chopped up in salads, or lightly steamed or baked. It is reputed to contain nutrients valuable to the body in restoring health to the urinary system. Class: *starchy vegetable*.

Lettuce: aster family. A good source of calcium, iron, potassium and phosphorus, the green outer leaves of lettuce are also rich in chlorophyll. All are essential biological requirements of the body during arthritis recovery and for maintaining health afterwards. Loose-leafed lettuce, such as Romaine and Bibb varieties, are nutritionally superior to the tight-packed Iceberg variety. Class: *green vegetable*.

Lychee. Also called the litchi, this nut-like fruit grows in Southern California and Florida. Lychees are best eaten fresh but are also available dried, when they taste like raisins. Fresh lychees are often mixed in with tropical fruits while dried lychees can be soaked and boiled for adding to vegetable casseroles or rice dishes. Class: *sub-acid fruit* (sweet fruit when dried).

Mamey. A russet-skinned tropical fruit found in South Florida and Mexico, the mamey has a dark-orange flesh rich in vitamins and minerals utilized by the body in normalizing carbohydrate metabolism. Class: *sub-acid fruit*.

Mango: cashew family. The large, oval varieties of mango now cultivated in South Florida rank among the most delicious and healthful foods in existence. The mango is ripe when slightly soft and when the skin turns yellow-red. Mango in the form of chutney or preserves has lost most of its nutrients. Class: *sub-acid fruit*.

Melons: gourd family. Their mildly diuretic effect makes musk melons such as the honeydew or cantaloupe helpful to the body in excreting gout-producing uric acid and other toxins. Chilled watermelon also makes a satisfying substitute for ice cream. Watermelon seeds may be beneficially chewed and eaten, or crushed and used to make a healthful herb tea. (Steep one tablespoon of the crushed seeds in a cup of hot water for one hour; then reheat and serve.) If you find that melons do not combine well for you with other fruits, simply eat melons alone. Class: *neutral fruit*.

Millet: grass family. Also called grain sorghum, cooked millet makes a satisfying breakfast cereal, especially when served with fruit. It may also be used in baking. Class: *cereal*.

Mushroom: yeast family. Though not always easy to digest raw, this edible fungi is a good source of vitamins and minerals. Try adding it to raw salads. If you have difficulty in digesting raw mushrooms, make them into a soup or use them in other cooked dishes. Class: *neutral vegetable*.

Mustard: cruciferous family. Cultivated (not wild) mustard greens add zest to a vegetable salad, or they may be lightly steamed. Eaten raw, mustard greens supply chlorophyll and other nutrients essential to the body in recovery from arthritis. Class: *green vegetable*.

Oats: grass family. This mineral-rich grain is probably the finest choice among breakfast cereals. Serve with *sub-acid* fruits such as apples, pears, peaches or with melons. Use only the coarse-cut oats sold in health food stores. Contrary to kitchen folklore, it can be cooked almost as quickly as "quick cooking" finely-chopped oats. Class: *cereal*.

Okra: mallow family. Okra's mucilaginous content is soothing to the digestive tract, and it can be cooked in a very brief time. Okra is delicious when baked with tomatoes, garlic and onions. Class: *green vegetable*.

Olive: olive family. Due to chemical additives, salt and processing, pickled olives have little nutritional value. However, cold-pressed olive oil is an acceptable dressing for salads and other foods, especially when mixed on a one-to-one basis with lemon juice. Mediterranean people claim it aids digestion and prevents constipation. Use olive oil only when fresh.

Onion: lily family. Chives, leeks, scallots, scallions, etc., can be eaten raw and enhance the flavor of any vegetable salad. Large yellow or white onions can be cooked or steamed with other vegetables, or made into an onion casserole. Class: *green vegetable*.

Papaya: pawpaw family. This melon-like tropical fruit ranges up to the size of a football. Peel to eat. In the hollow center of the orange-colored meat are scores of black seeds rich in the papain digestive enzyme. Papayas are ripe when the green skin is streaked with yellow. They are a good source of vitamin C and potassium and, if the seeds are chewed, of papain. The papaya is one of the great tropical fruits. The best are grown in Florida and Mexico, but smaller varieties from Hawaii are carried year around in many supermarkets. The papaya blends well with other sub-acid fruits. Try sprinkling it with lime juice. Class: *sub-acid fruit.*

Parsley: parsley family. This herb is rich in vitamins and minerals in which many arthritics are deficient. Chopped parsley should be liberally used in flavoring salads and other vegetable foods. Parsley can also be juiced or made into an herb tea. As either juice or tea it is mildly diuretic. Eaten raw, it supplies the body with nutrients utilized in excreting toxins. Class: *green vegetables.*

Pea: legume family. Fresh garden peas, especially edible pod varieties, combine fiber, protein, vitamins and minerals in a single delicious food. Mix them into vegetable salads or eat them alone as snacks. Dried peas, including lentils, are second choice but are still a good source of vegetable protein. If you must cook peas, do so for as brief a time as possible. Pea or lentil soup containing carrots, rice, celery, onion, potato, tomato and garlic is a tasty, nutritional meal. Class: *green vegetable.*

Peach: plum family. Peaches and nectarines are easily digested and supply important nutrients that the body requires to recover from arthritis and stay healthy. Peaches blend well with other sub-acid fruits; fresh (not canned) peach halves also taste good with cottage cheese. Dried peaches, if free of preservatives, are rich in minerals; they can be lightly stewed and served as compote. Class: *sub-acid fruit.*

Peanuts: legume family. Actually a bean, the peanut is an important source of energy and protein together with potassium, calcium, phosphorus, iron and unsaturated fat. Freshly-made peanut butter or cold-pressed, unrefined peanut oil retains most of the peanut's nutrients. If not kept refrigerated, both butter and oil will soon turn rancid. Try spreading peanut butter on celery sticks and use as a snack or as refreshments at a party. Class: *protein.*

Pear: apple family. A desirable, low calorie fruit, the pear blends well in fruit salads and may be cut and served on breakfast cereal. Leave the skin on if possible. Dried pears are acceptable only if free of preservatives. Class: *sub-acid fruits.*

Pecan: walnut family. This valued protein food is also a good source of calcium, phosphorus, potassium and unsaturated fat. It can be eaten with salads or as a snack. Class: *protein*.

Pepper: nightshade family. A rich source of Vitamin C when eaten raw, the green pepper enhances the taste of any vegetable salad. It may also be stuffed with cabbage, carrots and tomatoes and lightly baked. Hot peppers are not recommended. Class: *green vegetable*.

Persimmon: plum family. This reddish-orange fruit comes in light- and dark-skinned varieties. The dark-fleshed fruit may be eaten before it is actually ripe, but light-fleshed persimmons are astringent until perfectly ripe. Class: *sweet fruit*.

Pine nut: conifer family. Called pinon or pignola nut in its native Southwest, the pine nut is widely available in most health food stores. Although rich in protein, it is easily chewed and goes well with vegetable salads. Since they soon spoil, pine nuts should be kept refrigerated. Class: *protein*.

Pineapple: pineapple family. Imported from Hawaii, Puerto Rico and Mexico, the pineapple is readily available throughout the year. Its rich juice and fiber give the pineapple special nutrient values essential to the body in reversing arthritis or gout. Fresh pineapple juice is also a healthful beverage. Canned pineapple or pineapple juice should never be eaten. Fresh pineapple is delicious on breakfast cereal. Class: *acid fruit*.

Pistachio nut: cashew family. Unless purchased from health food stores, most pistachio nuts have been denatured by roasting, dyeing and salting. They are a fine source of protein, unsaturated fat and energy. Class: *protein*.

Plum: plum family. The numerous varieties of plum are all healthful foods. Prunes are dried plums and are a good natural laxative. Prunes can be soaked overnight and eaten without stewing or boiling. Class: *sub-acid fruit* (prunes are sweet fruits).

Pomegranate. Despite its tough skin and seed-filled pulp, the pomegranate contains nutrients beneficial to the body in excreting toxins. To eat this fruit, knead and squeeze it until soft. Then cut a small hole in the skin and suck out the pulp. The pomegranate may also be juiced. The juice blends well with carrot or apple juice. Class: *acid fruit*.

Potato: nightshade family. High in potassium, this starchy tuber is mainly an energy source. Bake lightly or cut and steam till tender. Class: *starchy vegetable*.

Pumpkin, marrow and squash: gourd family. Including winter and summer squash and zucchini, this large variety of starchy, gourd family vegetables supply abundant potassium. Softer varieties like zucchini can be eaten raw; others must be steamed or baked. They provide essential nutrients used by the body in restoring health to the urinary and circulatory systems. Eaten raw, or hulled and roasted, pumpkin seeds are rich in nutrients needed by the body when restoring the prostate to healthy condition. All these vegetables are delicious when lightly baked with tomatoes and garlic. The traditional pumpkin pie should be made with only whole wheat flour without fat or sugar. Class: *starchy vegetable.*

Radish: cruciferous family. Small, young radishes add zest to salads. (Large, older radishes become tough and fibrous.) Radishes are a healthful food only when not too pungent or "hot" to be eaten alone. They are mildly diuretic and their high fiber aids in preventing constipation. Class: *green vegetable.*

Raspberry: rose family. These small red, black or purple berries grow wild in many northern areas and at higher elevations elsewhere. They provide nutrients utilized by the body in restoring carbohydrate metabolism. Class: *sub-acid fruit.*

Rhubarb: buckwheat family. Very lightly cooked rhubarb is a good source of calcium and potassium and aids in cleansing the lower intestines and bowels. Owing to its oxalic acid content, rhubarb should not be eaten too frequently. Prepare it by placing cut rhubarb stalks in a pan of boiling water and removing immediately from the stove. Let stand a few minutes until ready. Do not allow rhubarb to become soft or mushy. Class: *green vegetable.*

Rice: grass family. Only unpolished (unrefined) brown or wild rice should be eaten. Organically grown long or short grain varieties are available inexpensively in most health food stores and granaries. Although rice is primarily a starch food, it is a good source of several B-vitamins and its high fiber speeds digestion and cleanses the bowels. This makes it very desirable in arthritis reversal. Prepare rice in a double cooker or simmer in a bean crock. Mix one cup of rice with 2½ cups of water until the rice rises and the water disappears. Most people overcook rice, thus reducing its nutritional value. Class: *cereal.*

Rutabaga: cruciferous family. Often called a Swedish turnip, this starchy root vegetable is a good source of calcium and calories. Steam briefly mixed with potatoes and other vegetables. Class: *starchy vegetable.*

Rye: grass family. Cooked cracked or whole rye forms a

good breakfast cereal, or it can be eaten with vegetables. Rye flour is also used in baking. Class: *cereal*.

Sesame seeds: pedalium family. Rich in calcium, minerals and protein, sesame seeds rank with sunflower seeds as one of the most nutritious and healthful foods. Sesame seeds mix well with sunflower seeds in a ratio of about four parts sunflower seeds to one part part sesame seeds. An oily butter called tahini is made from sesame seeds and, when fresh, is a fine, health-building food. Likewise, fresh, cold-pressed sesame seed oil is acceptable for cooking. Class: *protein*.

Spinach: goosefoot family. The several varieties of this green leafy vegetable supply a number of key nutrients needed by the body for arthritis recovery. Spinach is best chopped and added to salads, or it may be very briefly cooked. Most people overcook spinach, thereby releasing its oxalic acid which tends to leach calcium from skeletal bones. Class: *green vegetable*.

Strawberry: rose family. Like the cherry, the strawberry has proved beneficial in helping the body heal itself from gout and arthritis. Class: *acid fruit*.

Sunflower seeds: aster family. So rich are sunflower seeds in protein, calcium, iron and Vitamins A, E and the B-complex that many nutritionists consider them almost essential for bodily healing. Eat them alone or with sesame seeds and flavor with raisins. They can also be eaten with citrus or with vegetable salads. Freshly-prepared sunflower seed oil, butter and flour retain many of the key nutrients found in the seeds. Class: *protein*.

Sweet Potato: morning glory family. Primarily an energy source, the sweet potato and yam also contain an abundance of vitamins and minerals. They are best baked in their jackets but may also be steamed, grilled or casseroled. Class: *starchy vegetable*.

Tomato: nightshade family. Although acidic, the tomato becomes alkaline after digestion and, therefore, helps reverse acidosis in the body. As a result, it plays a key role in supplying the body with nutrients used in healing. Tomatoes are best picked when ripe as commercial tomatoes are picked green and never achieve the flavor or juice content of homegrown ones. Tomatoes combine well with protein or green vegetables and are best eaten raw in salads or in sandwiches. They can also be stewed, broiled, baked or made into soup. Class: *acid fruit*.

Turkey: turkey family. Light-colored turkey meat yields ten times as much whole protein as fat and is also a good source of phosphorus and potassium. Class: *protein.*

Turnip: cruciferous family. Both white and yellow varieties may be grated and eaten raw, or they can be lightly steamed, baked or used in soup. Turnip greens are valuable sources of Vitamin C and calcium and other nutrients required by the body in restoring health. Class: *starchy vegetable.*

Walnuts: walnut family. The several varieties including butternut and black walnuts are all good sources of protein, calcium, phosphorus, potassium and unsaturated fat. Walnuts supply the body with nutrients utilized in normalizing carbohydrate metabolism. Class: *protein.*

Watercress: mustard family. This crisp, peppery-tasting leafy vegetable is rich in vitamins and calcium and supplies a variety of nutrients essential to the body's healing powers. Add it to salads or use in sandwiches along with cucumber, tomatoes and alfalfa sprouts. Class: *green vegetable.*

Wheat: grass family. Cooked cracked wheat or wheat berries make an enjoyable breakfast cereal while whole grain wheat flour may be used for baking. While bleached or refined wheat flour, including any products made from white flour, is totally devitalized, whole wheat is a good source of fiber, iron, phosphorus and B-vitamins. Due to its tendency to form acid after digestion, wheat should be eaten sparingly. Class: *cereal.*

Yeast: yeast family. One tablespoon of brewer's yeast supplies 3.9 grams of protein, 21 grams of calcium, 175 mgs. of potassium, 23 mgs. of magnesium, 1.7 grams of iron and several B-complex vitamins. Unless you are allergic to it, brewer's yeast is a fine health-building food. Class: *protein.*

Yogurt, low fat: bovid family. One cup of low fat yogurt supplies the following percentages of U.S. recommended daily allowance: whole protein 30 percent; riboflavin 30 percent; calcium 40 percent; Vitamin B_{12} 20 percent; and phosphorus 35 percent. Low in fat but high in energy, low fat yogurt supplies many essential nutrients required for bodily healing. Eat it alone, with bread, or with salads or other foods. Class: *protein.*

Zapote: plum family. The brown, black, yellow and white varieties of zapote are fruits of Mexico and are all high in nutrients required by the body in reversing arthritis. Several varieties are now grown in South Florida. The black zapote is filled with a soft, dark flesh that resembles cream and can be eaten with a spoon. It can be used as a creamy dressing on fruit salads. All zapotes, in fact, can be blended and used as cream or as desserts. Class: *sweet fruit.*

INDEX

A

Acid, stomach (*see* Stomach acid)
Addictions:
  to allergenic foods, 78–79, 85–100
  to caffeine, 145
  to nicotine, 83
Additives, chemical, 145
Alabama, University of, Medical School, 16
Alcohol, 145
Alfalfa, 165, 192–193, 227
Allergenic foods, 56, 58–59, 85–100
  addictions to, 78–79, 85–100
  most common, list of, 90–91
  cutting out, 60–61, 94–95, 109
  cyclical allergens, 94, 211
  eating safely again, 94, 210
  fixed reaction allergens, 94, 211
  food families,
    cross-sensitivity to, 105–107
  identifying basic suspected foods, 85–100, 101–110, 117–118, 120, 123, 125–126
  identifying through reading, writing, 102–105
  preparing for food tests, 98–99, 115–116
  rotation diet, 210–214
  self-testing, food elimination test, 124
  self-testing, kinesiology, 119, 121–124, 127
  self-testing, pulse test, 111–120, 127
  self-testing, self-purification technique, 89–93, 95–110

Allergenic foods (*cont.*)
  self-testing, for sensitivity to, 73
  symptoms that identify, 101–110, 117–120, 122–127
  sensitivity to, variation with time, 93–94
  withdrawal symptoms from, 78–79, 86
Allergic response, 56
Allergy:
  to arthritis-causing foods, 33, 58–59, 85–100
  cyclical, 94, 211
  developing new, 130
  fixed, 94, 211
  hidden or masked, 56, 86–87, 90
  immuno-allergy, 56
Alternate-eating program, 204, 207
Alternative Diet Book, 132
American College of Allergists, 16
American Medical Association, Journal of the, 174, 181
Ankylosing spondylitis, 42–43
  recovering from, 92–93
  susceptibility difference in sexes, 49
Annals of Allergy, 16
Antibodies, 55–57
Antigen, 55–57
Anti-malarial drugs, 24
Applied Nutrition, Journal of, 186
Arthritic disease, 15, 41
Arthritis:
  articular, 41
  drug-caused, 17, 44
  how caused, 57
  non-articular, 41, 82
  not a medical problem, 21